W9-DCN-114

Marie Weil
Editor

Community Practice: Conceptual Models

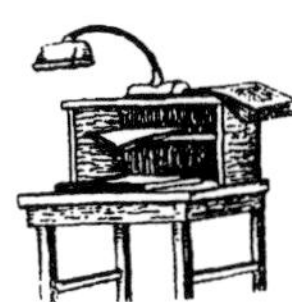

Pre-publication
REVIEWS,
COMMENTARIES,
EVALUATIONS . . .

This thoughtful book brings together some of the best new conceptual models for community practice.

It provides historical perspective on the changing context of theory and practice, presents major models and methods for knowledge development and action taking, and identifies unanswered questions and unresolved issues for future work. . . .

The authors are among the leading scholars and educators, each highly experienced, deeply committed, and anxious to communicate. The book will win an appreciative audience of organizers and planners, community activists and citizen leaders, in addition to students, scholars, and teachers in several social sciences and professional fields.

Professor Barry Checkoway, PhD
Professor, School of Social Work,
The University of Michigan

More pre-publication
REVIEWS, COMMENTARIES, EVALUATIONS . . .

In what is destined to be a much-heralded edited text, Marie Weil reaches long and wide in examining classic and new conceptual models for community practice. The editor convincingly argues that understanding the similarities and differences in the ways that models of community practice are conceptualized enhances the practitioner's ability to make the transition from theory to practice. . .

This comprehensive and well documented edited volume makes a significant contribution to community practice and theory development. It should be a welcomed resource for human behavior and macro social work faculty particularly on the graduate level. Practitioners, agency heads, students (masters and doctoral) and researchers should also find that the text is beneficial as it raises community practice to a new level of specificity. . . . I highly recommend this volume to schools of social work in the U.S. and throughout the world.

Moses Newsome, Jr., PhD
President, Council on Social Work Education, and Dean of the School of Social Work, Norfolk State University

* * *

Marie Weil's book, *Community Practice: Conceptual Models*, makes a major contribution to the literature on community social work practice. The book's emphasis on theory is not only designed to help students understand the conceptual basis of community social work, but it will also clarify many issues for practitioners and provide a better understanding of the ideas underlying community intervention.

The book examines and extends Rothman's well-known models of community intervention by examining these models with reference to current practice realities, feminist theory, international perspectives and further theoretical development. Weil's introductory chapter on the historical development of theory in community social work practice is the best written to date. Rothman's own chapter provides a fascinating insight into how a major figure in the field has revised and extended his original ideas. The international and feminist content is of a high quality.

The book should be required reading for all social work students. It is also highly recommended for practitioners interested in examining the conceptual basis of community social work practice.

James Midgley, PhD
Professor of Social Work and Associate Vice Chancellor for Research, Louisiana State University

Community Practice: Conceptual Models

ALL HAWORTH BOOKS AND JOURNALS
ARE PRINTED ON CERTIFIED
ACID-FREE PAPER

Community Practice: Conceptual Models

Marie Weil, DSW
Editor

The Haworth Press, Inc.
New York • London

Community Practice: Conceptual Models has also been published as *Journal of Community Practice,* Volume 3, Numbers 3/4 1996.

Cover design by Donna M. Brooks

The Haworth Press, Inc., 10 Alice Street, Binghamton, NY 13904-1580 USA

Library of Congress Cataloging-in-Publication Data

Community practice : conceptual models / Marie Weil, editor.
p. cm.
Includes bibliographical references and index.
ISBN 0-7890-0024-5 (alk. paper)
1. Social service. 2. Community development. 3. Community organization. I. Weil, Marie, 1941- .
HV40.C627 1996
361.8–dc21 96-47979
CIP

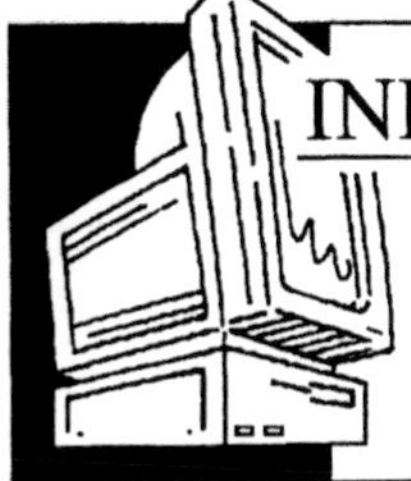

INDEXING & ABSTRACTING

Contributions to this publication are selectively indexed or abstracted in print, electronic, online, or CD-ROM version(s) of the reference tools and information services listed below. This list is current as of the copyright date of this publication. See the end of this section for additional notes.

- ***Alternative Press Index,*** Alternative Press Center, Inc., P.O. Box 33109, Baltimore, MD 21218-0401
- ***Applied Social Sciences Index & Abstracts (ASSIA) (Online: ASSI via Data-Star) (CDRom: ASSIA Plus),*** Bowker-Saur Limited, Maypole House, Maypole Road, East Grinstead, West Sussex RH19 1HH, England
- ***caredata CD: the social and community care database,*** National Institute for Social Work, 5 Tavistock Place, London WC1H 9SS, England
- ***CINAHL (Cumulative Index to Nursing & Allied Health Literature, in print, also on CD-ROM from CD PLUS, EBSCO, and SilverPlatter, and online from CDP Online (formerly BRS), Data-Star, and PaperChase (Support materials include Subject Heading List, Database Search Guide, and instructional video),*** CINAHL Information Systems, P.O. Box 871/1509 Wilson Terrace, Glendale, CA 91209-0871
- ***CNPIEC Reference Guide: Chinese National Directory of Foreign Periodicals,*** P.O. Box 88, Beijing, People's Republic of China
- ***CPcurrents,*** ITServices, 3301 Alta Arden #3, Sacramento, CA 95825
- ***Economic Literature Index (Journal of Economic Literature) print version plus OnLine Abstracts (on Dialog) plus EconLit on CD-ROM (American Economic Association),*** American Economic Association Publication, 4615 Fifth Avenue, Pittsburgh, PA 15213-3661
- ***Family Studies Database (online and CD/ROM),*** National Information Services Corporation, 306 East Baltimore Pike, 2nd Floor, Media, PA 19063

(continued)

- ***Family Violence & Sexual Assault Bulletin,*** Family Violence & Sexual Assault Institute, 1310 Clinic Drive, Tyler, TX 75701
- ***Guide to Social Science & Religion in Periodical Literature,*** National Periodical Library, P.O. Box 3278, Clearwater, FL 34630
- ***Human Resources Abstracts (HRA),*** Sage Publications, Inc., 2455 Teller Road, Newbury Park, CA 91320
- ***IBZ International Bibliography of Periodical Literature,*** Zeller Verlag GmbH & Co., P.O.B. 1949, d-49009 Osnabruck, Germany
- ***Index to Periodical Articles Related to Law,*** University of Texas, 727 East 26th Street, Austin, TX 78705
- ***International Political Science Abstracts,*** 27 Rue Saint-Guillaume, F-75337 Paris, Cedex 07, France
- ***INTERNET ACCESS (& additional networks) Bulletin Board for Libraries ("BUBL"), coverage of information resources on INTERNET, JANET, and other networks.***
  - JANET X. 29: UK.AC.BATH.BUBL or 00006012101300
  - TELNET: BUBL.BATH.AC.UK or 138.38.32.45 login 'bubl'
  - Gopher: BUBL.BATH.AC.UK (138.32.32.45). Port 7070
  - World Wide Web: http://www.bubl.bath.ac.uk./BUBL/home.html
  - NISSWAIS: telnetniss.ac.uk (for the NISS gateway)

  The Andersonian Library, Curran Building, 101 St. James Road, Glasgow G4 ONS, Scotland
- ***National Library Database on Homelessness,*** National Coalition for the Homeless, 1612 K Street, NW, #1004, Homelessness Information Exchange, Washington, DC 20006
- ***Operations Research/Management Science,*** Executive Sciences Institute, 1005 Mississippi Avenue, Davenport, IA 52803
- ***Public Affairs Information Bulletin (PAIS),*** Public Affairs Information Service, Inc., 521 West 43rd Street, New York, NY 10036-4396
- ***Rural Development Abstracts (CAB Abstracts), c/o CAB International/CAB ACCESS . . . available in print, diskettes updated weekly, and on INTERNET. Providing full bibliographic listings, author affiliation, augmented keyword searching,*** CAB International, P.O. Box 100, Wallingford Oxon OX10 8DE, United Kingdom

(continued)

- ***Sage Family Studies Abstracts (SFSA),*** Sage Publications, Inc., 2455 Teller Road, Newbury Park, CA 91320
- ***Social Work Abstracts,*** National Association of Social Workers, 750 First Street NW, 8th Floor, Washington, DC 20002
- ***Sociological Abstracts (SA),*** Sociological Abstracts, Inc., P.O. Box 22206, San Diego, CA 92192-0206
- ***Transportation Research Abstracts,*** National Research Council, 2101 Constitution Avenue NW, GR314, Washington, DC 20418

SPECIAL BIBLIOGRAPHIC NOTES

related to special journal issues (separates) and indexing/abstracting

- ❑ indexing/abstracting services in this list will also cover material in any "separate" that is co-published simultaneously with Haworth's special thematic journal issue or DocuSerial. Indexing/abstracting usually covers material at the article/chapter level.
- ❑ monographic co-editions are intended for either non-subscribers or libraries which intend to purchase a second copy for their circulating collections.
- ❑ monographic co-editions are reported to all jobbers/wholesalers/approval plans. The source journal is listed as the "series" to assist the prevention of duplicate purchasing in the same manner utilized for books-in-series.
- ❑ to facilitate user/access services all indexing/abstracting services are encouraged to utilize the co-indexing entry note indicated at the bottom of the first page of each article/chapter/contribution.
- ❑ this is intended to assist a library user of any reference tool (whether print, electronic, online, or CD-ROM) to locate the monographic version if the library has purchased this version but not a subscription to the source journal.
- ❑ individual articles/chapters in any Haworth publication are also available through the Haworth Document Delivery Services (HDDS).

ABOUT THE EDITOR

Marie Weil, DSW, is Professor at the School of Social Work of the University of North Carolina at Chapel Hill where she serves as Director of the School's Community Social Work Program. Dr. Weil is the principal author of *Case Management in Human Service Practice* and co-editor of two books on family and community practice. She has been engaged in the development of the Association for Community Organization and Social Administration (ACOSA) from its inception. Her publications include articles and book chapters on women and community organization and women in administration, and on work with vulnerable populations including service coordination in early intervention, child mental health, and adolescent pregnancy. She has co-edited several special issues of *Administration in Social Work.* Dr. Weil is involved in research on grassroots organizations particularly domestic violence programs and has published a number of articles on community practice. She is the editor of the *Journal of Community Practice*.

Community Practice: Conceptual Models

CONTENTS

Introduction

Marie Weil, DSW

This publication provides an opportunity to examine the commonalities and differences in ways that models of community practice have been conceptualized. Models provide a framework to understand, analyze and assess practice. They are useful as guides for practice and as teaching tools. Models hold an intermediate place between concrete practice skills and theory. They move the abstractions of theory into formulations that can guide interventions. They give direction to methods and skills. They embody theory and illustrate the actions that put theory into practice.

Concepts represent ideas. They are often complex ideas that provide an understanding of a phenomenon, an experience, or an ideal. *Community* is a concept, *organizing* is a concept, *empowerment* is a concept. Concepts may have a general popular or cultural understanding, and also have a more specific definition in relation to a particular theory. They arise from a theoretical or research context and have ascribed meanings that are clearly related to social/cultural context. Concepts are critically important in theory building and research because they structure our thinking.

A conceptual model or framework is a way of putting together concepts or ideas. It provides a design for how to think about or illustrate the structure and interworkings of related concepts–a structure, a design, or a system. A conceptual model is intended to illustrate the operation of a theoretical approach, and to build or demonstrate knowledge. A conceptual model of social intervention

[Haworth co-indexing entry note]: "Introduction." Weil, Marie. Co-published simultaneously in *Journal of Community Practice* (The Haworth Press, Inc.) Vol. 3, No. 3/4, 1996, pp. 1-3; and: *Community Practice: Conceptual Models* (ed: Marie Weil) The Haworth Press, Inc., 1996, pp. 1-3. Single or multiple copies of this article are available for a fee from The Haworth Document Delivery Service [1-800-342-9678, 9:00 a.m. - 5:00 p.m. (EST). E-mail address: getinfo@haworth.com].

will illustrate the components of that intervention and their relationships, interactions and intended consequences.

Conceptual models of community practice illustrate the diverse ways that community practice is conceived and delineate both the central and subtle differences among models in relation to characteristics such as: goals and desired outcomes, change strategies and targets of change, primary constituencies, and focus or scope of concern. Intervention models will also often illustrate the primary roles and skills needed to undertake moving a model from thought to action. One of the chief uses of conceptual models in community practice is that they can knit together complex ideas from the social sciences and community practice theory and illustrate how these ideas can be combined in the actions of practice. In many ways, conceptual models are the "pictures that are worth a thousand words" in that they visually and simply illustrate the interaction of complex thoughts and organize and illustrate ideas in ways that can directly guide actions and interventions.

The conceptual models presented in this volume should be helpful guides for practice and teaching. The first article provides an historical analysis of the development of community practice models from the earliest beginnings of community work in the U.S., highlighting the differences in emphases and commonalities of purpose across nearly a century of intellectual and practical development. It concludes with a presentation of the eight models of community practice developed by Weil and Gamble in 1995.

Jack Rothman's article, "The Interweaving of Community Intervention Approaches" presents his reworking of the basic three models of community organizing conceived in the 1960s that have guided generations of community organization students and practitioners. This reframing presents the greater complexity of mixed models of practice and provides a new depth to the conceptualization.

In "Modelling Community Work: An Analytic Framework for Practice," Ann Jeffries presents a meta model for understanding community practice. She builds from Rothman's basic concepts and provides an overarching structure to analyze and select intervention strategies. Jeffries has had the opportunity to use this framework in teaching both in the U.S. and in the U.K. and has found it to be an heuristic tool.

Cheryl Hyde, who has frequently written about feminist organizing and organizations, provides a critique of Rothman's conceptual model from a feminist perspective. She illustrates the wide range of feminist community practice throughout the basic and mixed models framework conceptualized by Rothman.

British models of community work are presented by Keith Popple. These models provide an interesting contrast to the U.S. conceptions and provide an illustration that allows us to see more of the cultural context of both the British and American models presented throughout the volume.

The final paper, "Theory for Community Practice in Social Work: The Example of Ecological Community Practice," provides an excellent means to examine a single theoretical model in detail. Ray H. MacNair analyzes ecological theory and presents a model of community practice grounded in this specialized theory. While a number of the other model frameworks presented draw from a variety of theoretical bases to illustrate the distinctions in practice approaches, this paper presents a model derived from a specific theory. This elaboration is useful in illustrating how any of the other discrete models presented might be articulated and fleshed out with more intensive use and interpretation of their theoretical base.

The conceptual models presented in this book represent the state of the art of conceptual modeling in community practice. They offer challenges and indicate directions for practice, for theory elaboration and testing, and for research. It is hoped that they will be useful in analysis, in planning for interventions and in research on community practice.

Model Development in Community Practice: An Historical Perspective

Marie Weil, DSW

INTRODUCTION

Community practice encompasses the processes, methods and practice skills of organizing, planning, development and change (Weil, 1994). Organizing relates to bringing people together for the betterment of social conditions and for social justice in neighborhoods, communities, regions, nations, and the world. Planning involves a range of processes and technical methods from neighborhood service planning through interorganizational planning for service integration and resource allocation, to social policy planning and implementation from local to global levels. Development refers to the social, economic and sustainable development efforts to improve

---

Marie Weil is Professor of Social Work at the University of North Carolina at Chapel Hill and Editor of the *Journal of Community Practice*.

Address correspondence to: Marie Weil, School of Social Work, CB# 3550, UNC-CH, Chapel Hill, NC 27599-3550.

The author would like to acknowledge Thomas Watson and Lanya Shapiro for assistance in research and the literature identification process, Dee Gamble for extraordinary collaborative work in development of the current models conceptualization and coauthorship of "Community Practice Models," and to NASW for permission to use the chart from the 19th Edition of *Encyclopedia of Social Work*, 1995.

[Haworth co-indexing entry note]: "Model Development in Community Practice: An Historical Perspective." Weil, Marie. Co-published simultaneously in *Journal of Community Practice* (The Haworth Press, Inc.) Vol. 3, No. 3/4, 1996, pp. 5-67; and: *Community Practice: Conceptual Models* (ed: Marie Weil) The Haworth Press, Inc., 1996, pp. 5-67. Single or multiple copies of this article are available for a fee from The Haworth Document Delivery Service [1-800-342-9678, 9:00 a.m. - 5:00 p.m. (EST). E-mail address: getinfo@haworth.com].

the conditions of life and protect the environment particularly for vulnerable communities and populations in poverty. Change refers to social action and social change strategies ranging from educational campaigns, to coalitions focused on strengthening services or changing policy, to social movements to redress social injustice.

The rationale for adoption of the term *community practice* is the wide range of connotations given to the usual "umbrella term" of *community organization* during its evolution as a practice discipline. In some periods, *community organization* has been used almost exclusively to connote community level social planning and service integration, while in other periods it has principally signified grassroots organizing and social action. In most periods both major functions have been recognized but the mixed usage can create confusion. *Community practice* provides a conceptual and theoretical umbrella that embraces and elaborates multiple models which often share several common processes but which have different emphases in knowledge base, methods, and skills. The growth of theory, literature, and research demands a conceptual framework that can encompass all the major models and modalities of work with people in communities and interorganizational alliances to deal with and find solutions for social problems. *Organizing*, *planning*, *development* and *change* processes are all integral parts of community practice and provide a framework to clarify and elaborate models of practice. This paper examines the origins and evolution of models of community practice and presents eight basic models of current community practice: social and economic development, neighborhood and community organizing, organizing functional communities, program development and community liaison, social planning, political and social action, coalitions, and social movements. Each of these community social work models is directed toward positive social change.

Community practice is a fairly recent term that has the advantage of providing a conceptual umbrella for the range of practice approaches, orientations, and models that have emerged in this arena since the 1890s. Conceptual models for practice are major tools for analyzing and teaching. They provide a level of abstraction and simplification that assists in comparing interventions and selecting appropriate modes of action for particular situations. To understand where we are going in this arena of social intervention, it helps to know our roots and lineage from the prototypical approaches in the late 19th century to the models in use at the close of the 20th century. The need for excellence in community practice is likely to increase in all settings in the next century. This paper concludes with examination of current models of community practice defined and elaborated by their major function and focus.

In an article in the 19th Edition of the *Encyclopedia of Social Work*, Weil and Gamble argue that current models of community practice have evolved from the earliest traditions of work with communities: the Settlement movement, the Charity Organization Society movement and the Rural Development movement (1995, p. 577). The Labor movement and the organizing and development histories of ethnic and racial groups likewise have made major contributions to the development of community practice models (Betten & Austin, 1990b; Rivera & Erlich, 1992). While there is still considerable work that needs to be done to refine and interpret the theoretical base of each of the current models, their evolution is an important part of understanding community practice and a means to clarify the commonalities and differences between and among practice approaches.

As used here, a model is not intended to signify a "boxed in" isolated or fixed approach with impermeable boundaries. As Rothman has so aptly illustrated (1989 & 1995), given the needs of particular situations, models will be mixed and phased to be most effective in the current situation and stage of organizational or community development. Creativity and adaptability arise from the process of mixing and phasing; however, it is very useful to have a primary model in mind so you can know what is being mixed and or phased, and so that theory and research concepts as well as knowledge and research findings can be used to strengthen and refine practice interventions.

DEVELOPMENT OF PRACTICE APPROACHES AND MODELS

Community practice in the United States has experienced five major periods in the creation of approaches, method specification, and model development and has been influenced by a steady progression in the development of the literature. This evolution began with the development of basic approaches in the taproots of community practice: the Settlement Movement, the Charity Organization Society Movement, and in Rural Development.

The evolution of models is demarcated by the following emphases and periods:

1. The Proto-Models of the "Taproots" era–1890s-1910s;
2. Definitions and Practice Method development–1920s-1930s;
3. Practice Method Specification–1940s-1950s;
4. Articulation of Basic Models–1960s-1970s; and
5. Expansion and Specification of Models–1980s-1990s.

Since community practice is so action oriented, it is not surprising that practice approaches and methods were developed and tested in the field and then written about. At each of the five stages, community practice has combined (a) the current knowledge base of relevant social sciences, (b) a value base grounded in social justice and democratic participation, and (c) practice methods and practice theory and guidelines. Much of early practice theory and conceptual development has evolved from practitioners' experiences and case studies written by practitioners and applied researchers. Throughout this evolution, community practice approaches, methods and conceptual models were developed to train and guide practitioners and students after they were tested through "trial by fire" in the field.

PROTO MODELS: THE TAPROOTS OF COMMUNITY PRACTICE–1890s-1910s SETTLEMENTS, CHARITY ORGANIZATION SOCIETIES, AND RURAL DEVELOPMENT

The Social Settlement Movement: Roots of Community Development, Planning, Organizing and Change

The Social Settlement Movement provided essential leadership for social change related to support for and inclusion of new immigrant communities, economic and social development, and combined physical and social planning to build stronger communities. It was widespread and diverse. For purposes of this presentation, the work of Jane Addams and the staff of Hull-House in Chicago are used as an exemplar of Settlement practice in and with communities. The most progressive settlements rapidly moved from planning for these communities to planning with residents for social and economic development and to combined physical and social planning strategies to build stronger communities. The book *Hull House Maps and Papers* (1885)–surveys, research, methodologies and findings–developed by Jane Addams, Florence Kelly, Julia and Edith Abbott, and other settlement residents, formed the basis of methods for studies of urban areas and the subsequent intellectual and methodological development of the Chicago School of Sociology, which has had a major effect on the disciplines of sociology, planning and social work (Deegan, 1990). This pioneering work developed methodologies and set a standard for community research as well as planning and development practice. The social work research model developed at Hull-House is very different from the sociological community studies which viewed the community or city as a laboratory–Addams and her colleagues conducted the research process so that residents were involved in the research and analysis and results were used primarily in extending community education and planning community-based action projects (Deegan, 1989). Major models of community work in organizing, planning, and development evolved from the Settlement Movement and have had incalculable impact on community practice and services in the non-profit sector. At their best, the settlements engaged and continue to engage neighborhood residents in educational reform, environmental actions, program development, inter-group relations, and broad arenas of social and economic development.

Model Development in the Early Literature

In her numerous publications and public and university lectures throughout the nation, Jane Addams consistently advocated for citizen participation. In her work she and her colleagues developed and enabled this process. The longer she worked at Hull-House, the more she separated herself from the more paternalistically-oriented settlement leaders and focused on the issues related to adult education, community-based planning and research and social and political action. Her vision was one of radical democracy–grounded in the belief that all people are equal and focused on actions to build equality in social, political and economic arenas. She was a staunch supporter of woman's suffrage, was an early feminist, engaged in the Labor Movement and was one of the earliest proponents of adult education and involvement of citizens in community problem solving. From her perspective, people in industrial areas needed information and knowledge about their situation and they needed to learn how to use information to change their social, political and economic conditions (Addams [cited in Lasch], 1965). She was committed to research, citizen participation, organizing and action to achieve a more democratic society.

While she worked closely with her colleague Florence Kelley, who had studied with Engels and other socialists in Europe and shared important points of the socialist vision, with her Addams separated from the Marxist perspective over the issues of means and ends, materialism, the conflict model and the status of women. She recognized that society was grounded in both conflict and cooperation, but held that if the ultimate goals of society were cooperation and peaceful relations, then the means to reach those ends needed to be congruent with the ends themselves (Addams, 1895; Deegan, 1990).

Charity Organization Societies: The Roots of Service Coordination, Community Planning and Interorganizational Relations

The Charity Organization Societies (COS's) established a new model and means to examine, develop, and support services for vulnerable populations and strengthen the planning, operations and funding base for the non-profit social welfare sector. These organizations grew out of and are grounded in volunteer leadership in planning and coordinating services in local communities. Stephen H. Gurteen's landmark publications laid the initial groundwork for coordinated planning and funding for community services in the nation with a strong focus on volunteer leadership. His "Beginning of Charity Organization in America" in *Lend a Hand* (Gurteen, 1894) translated British models for American application, while his

Handbook of Charity Organization (Gurteen, 1882) provided the blueprint for development of COS's throughout the nation. The extraordinary strength of the voluntary sector in this nation and its focus on coordinated planning and funding among agencies derives from this early work and its later incarnations in Community Chests and Health and Welfare Councils. These councils, which evolved into the United Way Movement, Jewish Federations, and other types of planning councils and alternative funding agencies such as the Black United Way and Women's Ways and planning councils have remained, in many communities, the major service coordination effort in the voluntary sector. There has been a recent revival in human service Planning Councils focused on service system development, service integration and interagency collaboration to serve communities.

While professional staff carry technical responsibilities for planning and coordination efforts, these coordinating planning bodies depend on volunteer leadership in review, recommendations, and decisions, and the board members of participating agencies as well as board members of the federated planning and funding groups are deeply involved in resource development, planning, allocation and monitoring of community-based programs.

The Lane report (1939) which first codified the *method* of community organization within social work emphasized that Councils worked to organize resources to meet community needs and promote coordination among social welfare organizations (Lane, 1939). As Tropman has noted, the continual question of focus for such planning councils and federated funding groups has been "whose resources" will be used and "whose needs" will be acknowledged and responded to (Tropman, 1967, p. 151). The tension related to prioritizing needs and leveraging resources is perennial in federated funding organizations and interagency planning efforts. The risk of bias in favor of powerful organizations in the human service sector and the risk of greater emphasis on or representation of power elites interests in decision-making processes has long been recognized. Tensions between volunteers and staff in prioritizing needs and making decisions about allocations are frequent. Finding effective ways to strengthen the connections and communications between grassroots groups and planning/funding groups is an ongoing problem, especially in relation to grassroots groups efforts to gain attention and secure funding for emerging issues and underserved populations.

Rural Development: The Rural Roots of Locality Development and Self-Help

While most of the literature related to the early history of community practice focused on urban neighborhood work and service coordination, rural development was equally important in its impact on the nation and on model development in several disciplines. Rural Community Development can be traced deep in American history. In *Democracy in America* (originally published in 1835), DeTocqueville observed that during his research, he was consistently amazed by a quality that he thought particularly American. With any group of five or more Americans, he commented, they are almost inevitably organizing themselves to create some project or association (DeTocqueville, 1961). Rural survival often demands cooperation and many efforts in rural development have been related to electrification, access to clean water, creation of cooperatives, and development of basic services (from day care to volunteer fire brigades) and social support systems.

The original professional workers in rural community development just prior to and during the 1920s and '30s were agricultural extension agents working out of land-grant agricultural and technical colleges. Unlike the Settlements and COS's, the major impetus for rural development resulted from legislation and federal funding (Austin & Betten, 1990). Extension service specialists provided training in home and farm demonstration to develop more efficient agricultural technology. While agents entered rural areas as experts, they learned to use a low key "discussion method" as trainers and in leadership development. Grassroots organizers armed with knowledge and new approaches to issues ranging from cultivation methods to development of cooperatives worked on local projects and often translated and facilitated the collaboration between farmers and extension agents (Lord, 1939).

While in these earlier years African American farmers were largely ignored by extension programs, some Historically Black Colleges provided their own extension agents and many Black farming families worked with them or their churches in rural collaborative organization and community support. In the rural segregated South, the Black community worked to take care of its own through self-help and mutual aid (Franklin, 1965; Burwell, 1996).

In many areas of the country, Betten and Austin note: "Rural people became partners with the government in the selection, financing, and direction of local extension programs" (Betten & Austin, 1990, p. 97; see also Brunner, Sanders, & Ensminger, 1945). In some areas rural Community Councils were formed. In the 1930s many farming cooperatives for both selling and buying were formed and one report states that in 1933 approximately one third of American farmers belonged to at least one cooperative (Betten & Austin, 1990, p. 99).

The self-help emphasis has remained strong in rural development practice. The Highlander Center has remained since the 1930s a major training ground for both rural and urban citizen participation activists. In recent years much rural community organization has related to protection of the environment. There is an entire stream of literature based on community work in rural areas, recently represented in a major text edited by Christenson and Robinson (1989), and examples of rural organizing around environmental issues can be found in *Lessons from the Grassroots* by Bob Hall (1988). In all of these efforts citizen education, research and participation are the guiding forces for protection of rural lands and people.

Early Trends in the Literature and Model Development

In their valuable history, Betten, Austin, and their colleagues document major practice movements and landmarks and show how these early efforts illustrate the three models engrained in community intervention in the U.S. (Bettan & Austin, 1990; Rothman, 1979). They analyze examples of *locality development*–the Cincinnati Unit Experiment, the International Institutes, and the Community Center Movement; *social planning*–the emergence of social planning and physical planning in that era, and a Federated Philanthropy in a Jewish Community; and *social action*–the Conflict Approach: Saul Alinsky and the CIO, and the Catholic Worker Movement during the Great Depression. These movements are the experience out of which models to guide practice were developed and codified.

Mutual Support Among Immigrants and Communities of Color

Early experiences of prejudice and exclusion encountered by immigrant groups and by peoples of color have also shaped the development of community practice. Racism and prejudice have shaped organizing and development in oppressed and disadvantaged communities. European immigrants developed their own mutual support institutions. The difficult struggles of European immigrants should not be forgotten, indeed much of the labor tradition, and many aspects of socialist and radical approaches to social action have developed in this country out of the history of these groups.

For African Americans, group support was not only desirable but critical for survival. During slavery and after emancipation, many African Americans organized small and larger scale mutual aid societies and support systems and later agencies and programs to serve their community. Historically the Anti-Slavery Societies were instrumental in providing for survival and support of fugitives escaping slavery in the South. Many support and aid groups have been formed through the Black church; ministers and church members from earliest times through the Civil Rights Movement to the present have served as community organizers and developers.

This significant history has received scant attention in the mainstream literature of the social sciences and community theory and practice literature. Major theorists such as W.E.B. DuBois and E. Franklin Frazier pioneered in development of theoretical concepts to guide self-help and social action and to increase understanding of the particular history of African Americans. Later historians have documented not only the social and economic injustices facing Black families and communities, but more critically have documented the history and practice of race work–the rich and complex tradition that embraces self help, mutual assistance, community organizing and development and social action within the African American Community (Franklin, 1965; Branch, 1988; Carlton-LaNey & Burwell, 1996).

DEFINITIONS AND PRACTICE METHOD DEVELOPMENT–1920s-1930s DEVELOPMENT AND CLARIFICATION OF METHODS OF INTERVENTION AND IMPACT OF PROFESSIONALIZATION

During the decades of the 1920s and '30s, fairly rapid method development took place in community work and considerable energy was devoted to developing commonly shared definitions to guide professional intervention. Social work training programs that had functioned more on apprentice models, moved into university settings and focus was given not only to teaching emerging social science theory but to developing practice theory in community work in local areas and interagency coordination. This period brought a major emphasis on professionalization and concomitant efforts to assure that community work was defined as a bonafide part of the social work profession. Academic and practice leaders during this period worked diligently to develop literature and teaching methods to assure that structural approaches, community approaches to practice, and intergroup approaches be recognized not only as a legitimate, but also as a pivotal part of social work's mission. The focus on the developing method of community work was identified as the principal way to keep a social problem focus, to maintain an environmental focus, and to formulate intervention in terms of structural approaches. Writers of this period connected case to cause and articulated the relationships of individual needs to social (and community) problems.

Considerable writing was devoted to providing comparisons and classifications of concepts and activities that illustrated similar elements or comparable functions between community organizing, group work and case work. In an article examining the development of community organization literature, Meyer Schwartz noted that during the 1920s and '30s the conceptualization of community organization in social work practice was primarily concerned with defining the purpose of community organization, clarifying the nature of community, developing ways to describe and practice with "the community" as client, and articulating the similarities with and differences of community organization from casework and groupwork (Schwartz, 1965). Method development was a driving force in the profession–partly as a way to clarify and teach practice, and partly as an effort to define social work as a profession with discrete knowledge and practice methods. Within the profession, the effort was focused on defining and elaborating roles of workers, clarifying the relationships among community organization practice, social action, and administration and developing practice literature to support these types of interventions.

During this period, writers, practitioners, and faculty were responding to the effects of rapid industrialization on the urban economy and culture. A major mission of many of the scholars who defined and shaped practice methods was to carry forward the goal of reconstruction of the small community–rural as well as urban. Schwartz argues that these writers were engaged in developing an inclusive vision of social welfare and notes that these writers envisioned "initiating and sustaining a democratic process involving citizens and experts at the grassroots level–to make a viable, creative entity out of the whole community" (Schwartz, 1965, p. 177). Connecting back to Addams and the ongoing development of American Sociology starting with the Chicago School, much of the methodology of this period was grounded in the philosophy of Dewey and focused on adult education methods as well as on basic sociological concepts.

Austin and Bettan (1990) and Schwartz (1965) provide excellent analyses of the development of the community organization method during this period. They identify as particularly productive and influential thinkers: Jesse Steiner, Bessie McClenhan, Walter Pettit, Eduard Lindeman, and Joseph Hart. These seminal thinkers on method employed the knowledge base of contemporary theories of sociology and social psychology. McClenahan and Steiner envisioned the development of a "study-diagnosis-treatment" schema to use in community work that would both identify general community problems in American society and recognize the uniqueness of each specific community. This formulation, identifying both commonalities and uniqueness and the "study, diagnosis, treatment" process, forms an essential approach to community work with elements that have carried forward to the present time. Given that there was a simultaneous emphasis on development of the profession and clarification of roles during this period, all these writers expressed a central concern with the relationship (conceptually and practically) of the citizen to the specialist (worker). They were committed to community organization as an expansion of democracy and talked about a needed process balance in which professionals could provide information, knowledge, and direction but in which nonprofessionals (citizens that is) maintained control of decision-making in community work.

During the early 1920s Bessie McClenahan developed detailed manuals to assist organizers in the process of entering a community, establishing relationships with community members and agency boards and building public relations through the press (McClenahan, 1921). She was also interested in rural organizing and urged the "appropriation of federal and state funds for the creation of bureaus devoted to the stimulation of interest in agriculture, the improvement of farming and rural conditions, and the extension of expert service to the local rural communities" (McClenahan, 1922, p. 134). In *Case Studies in Community Organization* (1928), Walter Pettit examined practice issues such as the role of the organizer, analyzing the community, developing leadership and establishing priorities. Jesse Steiner emphasized social science approaches and wrote about the major foci and division of labor between councils of social agencies and neighborhood associations in an interactive process of citizen involvement in social change (1930). He also wrote about the increasing connections between rural and urban areas and argued for the need for comprehensive service systems (Austin & Betten, p. 29). Joseph Hart's book *Community Organization* was published in 1927; he focused on the development of processes of "community deliberation" and saw the organizer as responsible to "stimulate individual responsibility for the common good" (Austin & Betten, 1990, p. 26).

Eduard Lindeman is one of the best known of these early theorists. He was committed to the primary role of the organizer as training "individuals, groups and communities to solve their own problems" (Austin & Betten, 1990, p. 24). He published widely and his major work, *The Community: An Introduction to the Study of Community Leadership and Organization* (1921), was extremely influential in practice and education. He recommended the establishment of goals in citizens' groups through the discussion method and acknowledged that community practitioners would need considerable skill in mediating conflict over decisions on means to achieve goals. He was deeply committed to democratic community decision making and designed steps to facilitate that process; his influential article, "Democracy and Social Work," was published in 1949 (Lindeman, 1949).

During the 1920s the diversity of organizations in communities and competing agendas were recognized by community organizers. As Austin and Bettan (1990) point out, recognition of these differences prompted writing and practice strategies to build community collaboration and cooperation. Emphasis on problem analysis and variations on the "study-diagnosis-treatment" method were employed as a major means of reconciling differences and helping groups or competing agencies understand each other's perspectives. Indeed in 1924 Mary Parker Follett developed the concept of "psychological interpenetration," defined as a means to enable people of different socioeconomic backgrounds to understand each other's perspectives (Syers, 1995, p. 2585). The central operative concept concerning the worker's role in regard to intergroup differences was the worker as "enabler" who could assist in seeing that alternatives and differences were clearly laid out and then foster a process of identifying options that could lead to reconciliation and avoid win-lose or either-or approaches.

During the Great Depression of the 1930s community organization began to receive greater local and considerable national attention and recognition. Federations raised considerable contributions to fight the social problems resulting from mass unemployment. The scale of the problem required federal governmental intervention. "Government in part, recognized community organization methods by including the marshalling of community support, fact finding, public education, and the coordination of public and private agencies within the public welfare structure" (Austin & Bettan, 1990, p. 29). The Social Security Act of 1935 was most likely the first federal statute to use the term "community organizing." It also required "social and community planning in order for states to receive funds" (Austin & Bettan, 1990, p. 30).

During the late 1930s the National Conference on Social Work commissioned a study of community organization to ascertain its relation to the profession as a method of social work, to compare it to casework and groupwork as major practice methods, and to identify its knowledge and skill base. Robert P. Lane undertook the study, producing a report based on findings from discussion groups in six cities. Lane's report presented at the National Conference in 1939 legitimated the place of community organization as a method of social work practice. Through the study process, agreement had been reached on five major propositions: (1) the term 'community organization' refers both to a process and a field; (2) the process of organizing a community or some parts of it is carried on outside as well as inside the general area of social work; (3) within social work, the community organizing process is carried on by some organizations as a primary function, by others as a secondary function; (4) the process exists on local, state, and national levels and also between such levels; and (5) those organizations whose primary function is the practice of community organization do not as a rule offer help directly to clients (Lane, 1939, pp. 496-97).

Despite this beginning codification, no single definition had been agreed on by the members of the discussion groups. Lane noted varying definitions all centered on "mobilizing resources to meet needs, initiating social services, coordinating the efforts of the welfare agencies, and building a welfare program" (Lane, cited in Schwartz, p. 178). During the end of this period the greater practice emphasis was on social welfare agency integration and planning.

The 1939 Lane report noted the following secondary objectives to accomplish the major aims of the community organization method: (1) fact-finding for social planning and action; (2) initiating, developing, and modifying social welfare programs and services; (3) setting standards; (4) improving and facilitating interrelationships by promoting co-ordination between organizations, groups, and individuals concerned with social welfare programs and services; (5) developing public understanding of welfare problems and needs, social work objectives, programs and methods; and (6) developing public support of, and participation in, social welfare activities. This major work both legitimated community organization in the profession and raised issues and questions that occupied practitioners and academics for the succeeding two decades (Schwartz, 1965). This report has a major place in the history of practice approaches and model development because it legitimated community organization in the profession and established it as one of the three major methods of social work practice.

PRACTICE METHOD SPECIFICATION–1940s-1950s GRASSROOTS WORK AND COMMUNITY PLANNING: METHOD SPECIFICATION AND CURRICULUM DEVELOPMENT

During the 1940s and 1950s there was great growth in the literature on community organizing and major work in specification of the practice method of community organization.[1] Considerable practice emphasis was placed on continued development of Health and Welfare Councils, community planning, and grassroots organization development. Several major books provide solid method specification, and much of the current perspective was consolidated and formalized at the end of this period in the publication of *The Community Organization Method in Social Work Education* (Lurie, 1959) as Volume IV of the Council on Social Work Education's major Social Work Curriculum Study.

Social and economic conditions as well as theory development in the social sciences shaped emphases in practice and curriculum development. The Great Depression had prompted major structural social interventions to deal with massive unemployment and the need for economic supports for the poor. In the aftermath of World War II, there was rising recognition of the concept and reality of social problems, naming of central issues, and willingness to plan broader strategies in relation to issues such as urban blight, poverty, racism, juvenile delinquency, prevalence of mental illness, and lack of provision for the aged. As Perlman noted, considering the work of this period, social planning and community organization leaders, academics and practitioners had to respond to the scope of these problems and "recognize the inadequacies of [earlier] interventions" (Perlman, 1971). There was a concurrent ongoing struggle to clarify the distinctiveness of community organization (CO) practice and to provide conceptual approaches that included CO as a major method in social work practice and education. Method specification provided clarity and illustrated unifying concepts and approaches to community problems as well as utilized case studies to illustrate the diversity of types of community intervention.

At the beginning of this period, Robert Lane presented a second report at the National Conference of Social Work which identified four basic concepts of community organization: group development, intergroup relations, integration, and adjustment between resources and needs (Lane, 1940). Group development refers to the processes of helping groups work together and develop and carry out plans; intergroup relations carried forward a major focus on concern with how different groups (ethnic, interests, etc.) could come together to work for community betterment; and integration referred to finding ways for communities to better meet the needs of citizens. Also in 1940, Arthur Dunham provided a definition for the field: "To help people find ways to give expression to these inherent desires to improve the environment in which they and their fellows must carry on their lives" (Dunham, 1940, p. 180).

Two major foci of community organization were specified by McMillan in his description of worker's major functions: (1) to stimulate people to use their powers for the cooperative improvement of group life, and (2) to assist in the development of the process by supplying the technical services required (McMillan, 1945). Kenneth Pray's work in the late 1940s was to emphasize the generic aspects of social work methods, preserve a unified purpose for the profession, and clarify the connection of CO to other social work methods. However, he focused primarily on creating social relations, placed less emphasis on achieving outcomes, and tended to ignore the change and leadership functions CO workers could play (Schwartz, 1965).

In his work, Wilber I. Newstetter (1947) stressed the "enabler" role of the worker and in contrast to Pray held that workers and community members shared responsibility for both process and outcomes. He elaborated the literature on intergroup work, specifying types of intergroups and describing workers' roles to help develop group structure, facilitate process, and enable members to function effectively as representatives of their constituent groups. In further work on defining and specifying the method, Dunham (1948) stressed that CO involved a very wide range of diverse activities and methods (Schwartz, 1965, p. 182). He explained this diversity in nine categories of job specialization ranging from local planning to legislative promotion.

Specification of Approaches/Orientations to Practice

Murray Ross played a major role in specification of CO methods and development of theory-based literature for curriculum. *Community Organization: Theory and Principles* (1955) focused on processes of work and provided the first sophisticated use of a range of social science concepts as central features tied into achievement of goals of the CO process. As Schwartz points out, "When Ross selected social science concepts, it was with a view which postulated that method was codetermined by suggestive theories from the social sciences and by social work values" (Schwartz, 1965, p. 183). He envisioned CO processes with geographic and functional communities in varied environments ranging from agriculture, to education, and community development.

Ross specified three primary approaches (orientations) in community organization practice: *reform orientation*; *planning orientation*; and *process orientation* (which he saw as the heart of CO). He also emphasized that these approaches could occur in a merged single approach or in sequential stages (Schwartz, 1965). Although Ross (like Pray) viewed direct social action as outside of social work, his formulations provided excellent groundwork for Rothman and later model developers to build on. Ross' second book, *Case Histories in Community Organization* (1958) provided a strong curriculum/practice tool in its specification of workers' roles and activities in engagement with individuals and with community groups, illustrated through eleven detailed case studies of intervention in different types of communities with different types of problems. He carefully drew on current social science concepts and provided examples of distinctions in process steps and strategy development depending on whether the particular approach was beginning from a more grassroots orientation of helping a community to "identify and mobilize itself to deal with its own problems," or more of a social planning approach responding to lack of welfare services "to develop a team to plan and organize welfare programs" (Ross, 1958, p. 19). He emphasized that personal development is inhibited by barriers to active participation in society and that individuals and groups can thrive through active participation.

In 1958 Arthur Dunham published *Community Welfare Organization: Principles and Practice,* which detailed practice methods in community planning and service coordination. He affirmed the generic base of social work and particularly stressed CO's connections with group work process. In contrast to Ross and Pray, however, Dunham considered social action as a basic aspect of CO practice, as part of professional practice, and as "inextricably related to community organization" (Schwartz, 1965, p. 184). Harper and Dunham released *Community Organization in Action* in 1959, which dealt with organizing and interagency coordination and planning. Finally Violet Sieder discusses the connections and interactions between community-wide planning and local organizing and action in two publications (Sieder 1947; 1950). In "What is Community Organization Practice in Social Work?" she identified concepts generic across community, group, and case work and described CO as a unique method of equal importance in social work. Sieder held that CO was a direct problem-solving service "engaging human beings in the context of the interaction of groups and individuals and involving organizational patterns of group life" (Schwartz, 1965, p. 185).

In "Social Work Community Organization Methods and Processes" (1958) Genevieve Carter described CO as encompassing a wide range of activities, some of which she held were clearly typical of social work and some that were not unique to social work. She identified the elements generic throughout social work methods as: (1) social study and diagnosis; (2) assessing the strengths in the situation; (3) utilizing resources; (4) modification or change, and (5) evaluation. The characteristics particular to community organization (and not typical of other social work methods) she noted as CO's (1) task or goal centered orientation; (2) its use of supporting and auxiliary processes; and (3) its transformation of the generic social work process elements into a more complex process comprising: (a) a reconnaissance phase; (b) a social study or diagnostic phase, using a wide range of concepts; (3) a planning or developmental phase (including research); and (4) an implementation phase (Schwartz, 1965, p. 185). These writers contributed greatly to definition and explication of community organization as an approach to problem solving and as a clear and distinct method of practice.

CSWE Curriculum Study/Community Organization

The Council on Social Work Education published a massive curriculum study in 1959 directed by Werner Boehm including Volume IV: *The Community Organization Method in Social Work Education* (Lurie, 1959). This volume provided articles which defined community organization practice, articulated concepts, values and methods, and described teaching strategies for class and field. Harry Lurie served as the consultant for the CO volume and compiled and wrote the study. A panel of fifty-two noted experts participated in planning, organization and content development of the study. Lurie's study report provided chapters on: (1) the teaching and practice of community organization; (2) working definition of community organization as a method of social work; (3) basic concepts in educational objectives for co-practice; (4) elements of CO method in social work practice; (5) course content and field instruction and (6) summary comments. Position papers are presented in the CO study's appendix including ones focused on field work, theory, and methods and skills. Genevieve Carter provided the chapter on theory; Arnold Gurin formulated methods and skills related to work in national agencies; Arlien Johnson explained community organization roles and responsibilities in social casework agencies; Wayne McMillan provided a paper on teaching; and Violet Sieder outlined the tasks of the CO worker.

In their paper, Wilber Newstetter and Meyer Schwartz discussed the need for a foundation course in "community organization for social welfare" for all social work students connecting the basic methods, using the "study, diagnosis, action" approach, and focusing on issues of (a) intergroup work process, (b) administrative processes at intergroup and interagency levels; and (c) promotional and public education processes. They presented objectives and provided a curriculum outline for the recommended basic course. Their article identified concerns (that are still currently familiar) that the majority of social work students are not adequately connected to community, environmental, organizing, and policy issues and their course design was designed to remedy this problem and enable schools to turn out workers in all three methods who could engage with community issues.

In presenting a structure for a specialized community organization curriculum in social work, E. C. Shimp argued for a two year program that would encompass: "(1) the philosophy of social work; (2) both broad and specific knowledge of the social services; (3) dynamics of human behavior–individual, group, and community; (4) methods and skills; (5) administration; and (6) research" (1959, p. 236). He expressed three areas of special significance in preparing students for community organization practice, which are distinct from the concerns in preparing caseworkers and group workers because of the difference in the nature of clients for the three methodologies. The areas of special concern that he identified were: (a) philosophy and attitudes; (b) methods and skills; and (c) knowledge and understanding.

Shimp argued that community organization would include a variety of structures but be united by a common philosophical framework which he conceptualized as encompassing the following principles: "(1) the worth and dignity of the individual and faith in democratic processes; (2) the desirability of improving relationships among individuals, groups, organizations of people, neighborhoods and communities; (3) the right of individuals, groups and communities to differ but still retain a responsibility for the well being of others; (4) the ability of individuals, groups and communities to change; (5) the process of interaction as an instrument to effect change; (6) the right of self-determination; (7) that the end result cannot be divorced from the means; (8) that in a democracy, participation of people from all walks of life is essential in reaching appropriate decisions; (9) that a worker's self-awareness is an integral part of his performance and accomplishment; and (10) that an orderly process is essential and compatible with desirable change in value systems and social institutions" (1959, p. 238).

Methods and skills curriculum, Shimp argued, should prepare students to use the CO process–"a way of working on an orderly, conscious basis to effect defined and desired objectives and goals" to assist citizens of the community to:

1. identify, diagnose, and define community problems or needs;
2. ascertain appropriate factual data regarding the problem of need;
3. analyze the data, and determine their significance;
4. consider possible solutions and decide on the appropriate course of action;
5. set in motion actions determined by the community to be most likely to achieve the goal sought (Shimp, 1959, p. 238).

He identified the major skills areas needed by CO practitioners to be: "(1) relationships; (2) participation and representation; (3) leadership and its development; (4) authority and how it is derived in a democratic process; (5) use of one's self as an enabling or helping person; and (6) the fusing of the above into an acceptable way of working in moving from problem to solution (Shimp, 1959, p. 239). With regard to the intellectual base, Shimp stressed the need for more knowledge in relation to research and evaluation methodologies and the use of information and data as well as advanced knowledge in a variety of practice areas such as intergroup work, planning, administration and financing of services.

The Curriculum Study CO Volume illustrates the richness and diversity of practice developed by that time. This work forms a major milestone in the codification of community practice and education in social work. By the close of the 1950s, a substantial and wide ranging literature on community organization theory, practice (at local and national levels), and values was available to build upon in the resurgence of interest and opportunities for practice in the mid-1960s.

Other Developments During the Period

Aside from the directions described in the literature review, a variety of efforts related to community organization were occurring. Bettan and Austin (1990) discuss the Dorothy Day, Peter Maurin, and Catholic Worker Movement and its achievements in community work and programs to serve the most oppressed. Saul Alinsky, emerging from involvement with the CIO in the Labor Movement, translated those tactics into neighborhood organizing in the "Back of the Yards" area in Chicago. Alinsky epitomized the conflict model of social action. "Alinsky clearly adopted his general power-building approach and specific tactics from the CIO. . . . Thus, controlled conflict illustrates the intertwining of two aspects of community organizing: the building of activist CIO unions of the 1930's and the creation of Alinsky's militant people's organizations whose techniques grew out of the CIO experience" (Bettan & Austin, 1990, p. 161).

During this period Myles Horton provided another strong voice for community work and citizen participation. He developed the Highlander Center in Tennessee and established a place where adults of all races (Blacks and whites together in the South in the 1950s!) could come together, learn together, examine and research community problems and develop leadership capacities to take back to their homes. Horton's philosophy was grounded in adult education developed from the context, knowledge, and perspective of the people. The Highlander staff and its participants believed that leadership was a broadly, not narrowly, distributed quality and adopted Horton's maxim: "Learn from the people; start their education where they are" (Adams, 1985; Horton, 1990). Highlander's impact on community work, especially in the South, is incalculable. Rosa Parks and many lesser known community and environmental activists have participated in its programs. Numerous people who became leaders in the Civil Rights Movement of the 1960s received their training through Highlander, and in many ways that movement sets the tone for community organization and practice in the 1960s and '70s.

ARTICULATION OF BASIC MODELS–1960s-1970s LOCALITY DEVELOPMENT, SOCIAL PLANNING, AND SOCIAL ACTION

The era of the 1960s-1970s was marked by the second rediscovery of poverty in America (Harrington, *The Other America*, 1962), the Civil Rights Movement, the War on Poverty and the Vietnam War. These times of social upheaval and efforts to further citizen participation and social justice (before the Vietnam War consumed and conflicted the nation) catalyzed greater activism among faculty and students of social work and brought forth a focus in community practice that emphasized direct organizing for social justice issues, direct social action using a variety of strategies and approaches, and the development of advocacy planning as part of a way to bring power and knowledge to the people.

Social activism was a major thrust during the 1960s and the Civil Rights Movement and governmental anti-poverty programs encouraged a climate favorable to organizing, social action and change in public and voluntary sectors. From the mid-1960s through the 1970s, major writing, research and model development occurred. The growth in the literature during this period was astounding and its scope, unfortunately, cannot be presented here.[2] A major literature review of this period is called for, but the current paper can focus only on those aspects of literature development that focused on community organization model development. Jack Rothman's definitions, and formulation of three basic models of community organization, serve as the capstone of the earlier periods' development of practice approaches and orientations. Generations of students have been reared on his work. His models have in fact become the touchstone for community practitioners in the U.S. and in many parts of the world.

In 1967 Jack Rothman presented his seminal article on community organization models (Rothman, 1967). He identified, defined, and delineated three basic models: *locality development*, *social planning* and *social action* that have been the central point of reference in describing and analyzing subsequent decades of community practice efforts. In response to the times, he focused much attention on local planning, development and action efforts rather than on coordinated community service planning and gave little attention to organizing communities of interest. Rothman's recent revision and expansion of his typology is presented elsewhere in this volume; the current presentation only traces aspects of model development.

Social Planning Model

Rothman's codification of the elements in social planning identified the major goals as problem solving focused on substantive community problems utilizing a basic change strategy of fact gathering and rational decision making for a total community or a specified functional community. The practitioner roles emphasized technical skills in research, analysis, program implementation and facilitation. The client role was typically expected to be consumer or recipient.

Locality Development Model

Locality development had major process goals of self-help and community capacity building and focused on broad groups of people involved in determining and solving their own problems. This model usually focused on a small community with citizens participating in an interactional problem solving process. The practitioner role was primarily that of enabler-catalyst, coordinator, and teacher of problem solving skills.

Social Action Model

Rothman summarizes the elements of this model as including both task and process goals geared toward changing power relationships and basic institutions. Members of disadvantaged populations are the constituents of such groups with the practitioner functioning primarily as an activist advocate. Major strategies include contest or conflict to achieve goals.

Revision of Models: Mixing and Phasing

As Rothman (1987) discussed in his revision of the original article, these models do not typically exist in isolation. Transitions among development, action, and planning are common in a community process. He described such transitions as the mixing and phasing of models. Comparable to Rothman's perspective, the major works published in the late 1960s and '70s reflected the activist approach with most of the literature focused primarily on organizing or local planning activities. Work that related to interagency coordination, and much coverage of planning issues migrated to the growing literature on social administration. Jobs were available and literature was needed to support new and emerging practice efforts and to educate students for effective practice. That decade produced a wealth of community organization literature as jobs were available for organizers in anti-poverty programs, settlement houses and neighborhood centers and many other non-profit settings. Graduate programs multiplied and the literature burgeoned with more specified models, evaluation efforts, case studies and theory development. In a brief treatment of this era, justice cannot be done to the many writers who contributed greatly to this expansion of knowledge and refinement of practice approaches. This discussion can focus only briefly on the basic trends in this second major wave of model development.

Other Developments in the Literature

During this period, almost all community work was described as community organization. Following the major developments in the literature during this activist decade the literature has continued to grow despite an inhospitable political climate and the sharp downturn in the number of professional schools offering specializations in community organization and social planning. During this period, major texts were developed on community organizing–Brager and Specht (1973), Cox, Erlich, Rothman, and Tropman (4th edition, 1987); social planning–Lauffer (1978), Ecklein and Lauffer (1972), and Gurin and Jones (1970); social action–Saul Alinsky (1971), Kahn (1982); and development–Blakeley (1979), Christenson and Robinson (1989), Rubin and Rubin (1986).

The relative amount of attention to community oriented practice and increasing specialization are clearly evidenced in successive issues of the *Encyclopedia of Social Work.* The Fifteenth Issue published in 1965 included four articles on community development, organization, planning and development, and social action. The *Encyclopedia's* Sixteenth Issue (1971) featured five articles on community welfare councils, development, centers, organization and social planning, and social action. In the Eighteenth Edition (1987) twelve articles on "Citizen Participation," "Community-Based Social Action," Political Action in Social Work," "Civil Rights," "Community Development," "Community Theory and Research," "Macro Practice: Current Issues and Trends," "Planning and Management Professions," "Social Planning," "Social Planning and Community Organization," "Social Planning in the Public Sector," and "Social Planning in the Voluntary Sector" were provided thus tripling the articles focused on community practice. The increasingly specialized models reflected in this progression in *Encyclopedia* coverage have been confirmed in subsequent literature.

COMMUNITY PRACTICE: EXPANSION AND SPECIFICATION OF MODELS–1980s-1990s

During the 1980s and '90s models of community practice have expanded and the delineation of models has become more specified. Three major model frameworks have been introduced: (1) a five model framework in a book on theories of community social work edited by Taylor and Roberts (1985); (2) a major revision and expansion of his earlier three model schema by Jack Rothman (1995); and (3) an eight model framework for community practice developed by Weil and Gamble (1995). These efforts relate to and complement each other while each provides a different perspective for and analysis of models. In addition to this work on generic models, considerable work has been done on Feminist models and approaches to community work (Hyde, 1986, 1990, 1994; Weil, 1986; Brandwein, 1987) and approaches adapted by racial and ethnic groups (Daley & Wong, 1994; Rivera & Erlich, 1992; Bradshaw, Soifer & Gutierrez, 1994; Gutierrez & Lewis, 1994). All these developments have clarified the purpose and operations of specific models and with the increased specification particularly in the two 1995 presentations should facilitate assessment and analysis of practice situations and provide a more solid basis for case studies and comparative research across models and on practice innovations. The evolution, differentiation and specification of models in the 1990s has occurred because of adaptations in practice in response to the increased complexity of the social and economic environment. The following discussion illustrates the evolution of model specification during this period.

Five Models Framework: Taylor and Roberts

Sam Taylor and Robert Roberts edited and published *Theory and Practice of Community Social Work* in 1985. With support from a Canadian Foundation the group of authors was able to meet together in Saskatchewan to review and critique first drafts of chapters. The editors lamented the lack of well-formulated theories but concluded after a careful review of the literature that "distinct approaches do exist and that these can serve as a springboard for organizing more cogent conceptual frameworks that would be of value to practitioners and researchers" (Taylor & Roberts, 1985). They commissioned five chapters on models or approaches to community social work that will be detailed below and six chapters on specific arenas of community social work practice with: oppressed minority communities, the aged, mental health settings, health care, child welfare, and in Third World Countries. Taylor and Roberts provided an introductory chapter entitled "The Fluidity of Practice Theory: An Overview" and Carel Germain discussed "The Place of Community Work within an Ecological Approach to Social Work Practice" in a chapter which places community work within its professional context. In the chapter on the fluidity of practice theory, Taylor and Roberts provide an interesting analysis of the tensions between approaches to practice that are "sponsor determined" and those that are "client determined" (pp. 12-15). In this discussion they further develop issues discussed by Rothman in his original and adapted presentation of three models and particularly the discussion of tension between social planning and social action as discussed by Brager and Specht in their classic text *Community Organizing* (1973; pp. 171-212). Taylor and Roberts argue that models can be classified and understood in relation to the degree to which both sponsors and clients determine: "(1) the parameters of practice; (2) the alternative strategies that can be considered; and (3) the extent to which decisions are influenced by clients or sponsors" (p. 12).

Taylor and Roberts' book provides chapters comparable to Rothman's three basic models and provides two newly specified models. The basic models for community social work and their emphasis on either sponsor or client determination as presented in this book are:

- Program Development and Coordination: Fully Sponsor Determined
- Planning: Seven Eighths Sponsor Determined

- Community Liaison: One Half Sponsor/One Half Client Determined
- Community Development: Seven Eighths Client Determined
- Political Empowerment: Fully Client Determined

These basic models are described briefly.

Program Development and Coordination. Kurzman (1985) delineated and specified a model not explicitly covered in Rothman's typology but endemic in community work since its inception. Program development and service coordination is grounded in community work's oldest traditions: the settlements and charity organization societies. This model focuses primarily on implementation that may be carried out in the public sector, in private sector agencies serving a geographical area, in functional communities of interest, or by a federation or council of agencies.

Planning. In updating the social planning model, Rothman and Zald (1985) stress technical skills and research strategies based in rational planning models that are applicable at local, regional or national levels to conduct research, produce plans and forecast outcomes. Their treatment of planning theory in social work community practice reveals increased sophistication and builds on Rothman's earlier model. They discuss the beginning emergence of more transactive/people oriented efforts within social planning and more advocacy oriented, radically oriented, or clearly political approaches to planning that take more account of the expectation of sponsors or constituencies. They stress process skills: managing organizational processes, exerting influence, and conducting interpersonal relations; and technical or task oriented skills: designing, expediting, and implementing.

Community Liaison. Recognizing that in the 1970s and 1980s many social work agencies ceased to employ organizers and planners, Taylor (1985) describes a model not covered in Rothman's typology, the community liaison approach, which consists of community work functions carried by administrative and line staff of human service agencies. This model builds from earlier approaches utilized by direct service workers and administrators treated by Arlien Johnson and E. C. Shimp in the 1959 Curriculum Study (Johnson, 1959; Shimp, 1959). In this model, community practice is a secondary function to an agency's primary responsibility for direct service delivery. Administrators carry expected roles such as community relations, support activities, environmental reconnaissance, and interorganizational relations. With the growth of generic practice models, direct service workers may well be involved in client advocacy, needs assessments, and program development. Both administrators and direct service workers need community practice skills to work with consumer groups and to adapt their programs to target population needs.

Community Development. Lappin wrote about the community development model (Rothman's corollary is locality development) with a strong emphasis on enabling, leadership development, self-help, mutual aid and locally based community study and problem solving. The model places major stress on citizen participation and educational processes. Lappin had written and worked with Murray Ross on the Second edition of *Community Organization: Theory, Practice & Principles* (1967). He describes the roots of all community development practice in the enabling role. Lapin notes that Biddle and Biddle (1965, p. 82) "equate enabling with the role of an encourager whose involvement is most intense in the early stages and tapers off as the confidence and capabilities of the residents come to the fore"(p. 62). He argues with Smith (1979, p. 50) that the enabler role "(rather than that of the organizer) is the best practice approach if a community is to arrive at the point where it is able to judge its own needs" (p. 62). The enabler role can be used in both neighborhood development (direct community work) and in community welfare work (indirect community work). The primary focus that Lappin takes, following Ross, is on process emphasizing a range of generic skills and tasks: "(1) system maintenance; (2) planning activities; (3) developing enabling relationships; (4) mobilizing initiatives; (5) innovative tasks; and (6) educational and interpretive tasks" (p. 67). Lappin notes the shift in the 1960s from neutral enabler to partisan activist with a greater emphasis on a central role as advocate. He outlines community development in the Third World as still carried forward more through enabling processes and notes the increased advocacy focus in neighborhood development in the U.S. Finally Lappin describes commonalities but sees more divergences between community development and community welfare organization, except in the advocacy planning councils that were active in the 1970s.

Pluralism and Participation: The Political Action Approach. The political action approach described by Grosser and Mondros (1985) relates closely to Rothman's social action model (1967). Their presentation is grounded in conflict theory and the competition of diverse interests in a pluralistic society. Political empowerment is a clear focus and the intended outcome of citizen participation. As they note:

> One objective of community social work practice is to reduce the erosion of pluralistic democracy by ensuring and/or maximizing participation by citizens in the institutions and systems of society. A related goal is that of facilitating alternate channels of participation through the development of new organizations of the excluded. In both cases, a consequence of community practice is expansion of the quality and impact of participatory efforts. (1985, p. 155)

Grosser and Mondros discuss three types of change that occur with the political action approach: personal growth; acquisition of skills; and institutional and political accountability. Workers focus primarily on roles as educator, resource developer and activist. This orientation can be carried forward in either legally mandated organizations or self-generated organizations. They discuss a variation on phasing of models noting that groups such as neighborhood associations or minority rights organizations may develop alternative services for their communities of interest–the development of specialized AIDS/HIV service and support programs designed by the Gay and Lesbian communities are one example of this transformation. This approach clearly specifies social action as geared toward changes in political power. Grosser and Mondros emphasize four major strategies: (1) morale building for people and organizations using cooperative tactics; (2) problem-solving–developing new services, establishing new local decision-making bodies; instituting specific changes in an environment largely through collaborative tactics; (3) function transfer to build responsive services such as creating support networks or providing emergency benefits, or creating organizations such as community credit unions and cooperatives; and (4) power transfer–creating powerful counterveaning organizations at the community level usually requiring conflict strategies.

Taylor and Roberts hold that these five models are still fluid and in need of further theoretical development. One measure of difference they noted in 1985, is the relative level of sponsor versus consumer influence on decisions. In the current world of practice, however, there is increasing pressure to make all models more responsive to consumer/citizen perspectives. Indeed the mandate for consumer and citizen involvement increasingly comes from members of service populations, vulnerable groups, emerging functional communities, and disenfranchised communities. While these changes are sometimes discomforting to professionals vested in their own expertise, it is welcome to community workers who have traditionally been trained to work as partners with citizens in mutual planning, organizing, action and development processes. What is critical is to develop clarity in any program about the process of citizen participation and the locus and balance of decision making responsibility. Commitment to empowerment and citizen participation should be an element in all community practice models.

Feminist Analyses of Community Practice Models

While women have always been a part of general community practice, as leaders and participants (indeed the majority of members of neighborhood based organizations and projects have typically been women, and have always been involved in specific projects operated by women focused on women and children and social causes), feminist scholarship on community practice models is a relatively recent development. Certainly most of the women leaders in the Settlement Movement and many women leaders in interagency work as well were engaged in the first wave of American feminism and worked diligently for women's rights and opportunities. As Deegan (1990) has argued, the settlement movement and indeed the social work profession itself provided (along with nursing) some of the earliest opportunities for women in professions. Addams particularly was involved in cultural feminism and through Charlotte Perkins Gilman became more involved with radical feminist ideas (Deegan, 1990). Addams spent much time involved with working women, fought against the hypocrisy of male reactions to prostitution and supported the labor movement. In Chicago, women's labor unions were largely organized through Hull-House. As noted in earlier sections of this paper women have been leading practitioners and writers in much of community work.

The second wave of American feminism sparked a growing literature in the social sciences and social work. In 1986, in *Feminist Visions for Social Work* (Van Den Berg & Cooper), the chapter "Women, Community, and Organizing" noted that women have always been involved in general community organizing and increasingly in feminist organizing (Weil, 1986, 1995). In considering women as a community of interest, the chapter outlined frameworks and approaches arising from liberal, socialist, and radical political approaches and the emerging approaches of women of color in relation to the following model components: goals, assumptions about sexism and oppression, orientation to power, emphasis of change strategies, tactics, roles of change agents, and action systems.

The following feminist principles: (1) use of feminist values; (2) valuing of process; (3) consciousness raising and praxis; (4) wholeness and unity; (5) reconceptualization of power and empowerment; (6) democratic structuring; (7) the personal is political; and (8) orientation to structural change, grounded the chapter, which states that in feminist practice: (a) "*Goals* will always relate to the elimination of oppression; (b) *Power* will be conceptualized as facilitative, enabling, and shared within and among groups; (c) *Strategies* for change will stress the need for congruence of means and ends and will be grounded in egalitarianism . . . and mutual responsibility; and (d) *Action* will be based on feminist principles" (1995, pp. 128-130). The chapter provides brief descriptions of the five models described in Taylor and Roberts (1985) and presents a chart of feminist adaptations of those models incorporating feminist issues and roles.

Brandwein in 1987 provides a useful feminist chapter, "Women and Community Organization" in *The Woman Client.* She presents a brief historical background on women leaders and cycles of dominant professional orientation. She provides a gender analysis of Rothman's three basic models stating that both social action and social planning fit male gender stereotypes–social action as "macho" and social planning as "scientifically based, rational, and logical" (p. 115). During the 1960's she notes even neighborhood-based community organizing became tinged with a "definite anti-female cast." She notes that: "Moreover, the infusion of a social science theory base in community organization and planning introduced male-dominated disciplines such as economics, political science, and sociology. The men who had been recruited into social work in the 1950s became leaders of the conflict-oriented, social science-based community organization of the 1960s and recruited men into the profession and dominated the literature of the period (pp. 115-16). Brandwein emphasizes the following aspects of a feminist prism through which to view community organizing: androgyny, wholism, synergy, win-win power orientation, web of relationships, and egalitarian relationships. Both Brandwein (1987) and Weil (1986) discuss curriculum issues and implications related to feminist and nonsexist practice.

Other writers, notably Hyde and Gutierrez and Lewis, have furthered development of feminist approaches to community practice. Hyde has written about feminist organizations and organizing, developing typologies and models (see article in this volume; Hyde, 1994, 1991, 1990, 1986), while Gutierrez and Lewis have outlined a feminist approach and perspective on community organizing with women of color (1994, 1992).

Diversity and Community Organizing

Diversity has always been an issue of concern in community practice. The settlements and COS organizations both dealt with the poverty and needs of immigrants and members of racial and ethnic minorities. As noted earlier, a strong historical analysis and current practice literature is now being developed largely by members of ethnic and racial groups that have had to deal with social and political oppression. As historical analyses offer a corrective to noninclusive versions of history, so specialized perspectives on community development, organizing, planning and change offer a new richness to the current practice literature. Felix Rivera and John Erlich (1992) undertook their edited book, *Community Organizing in a Diverse Society,* because a book on organizing by and with people of color did not seem to exist. As they state "Racism–political, economic, and social–is at the core of the problem" (p.1). In the introduction to this first book focused on organizing within communities of color, Rivera and Erlich critique both conservative and liberal theoretical approaches as neglecting the primary importance of culture. They find a paucity of easily identifiable radical or progressive ideological positions in the ten chapters focused on different groups. What is clear, they suggest:

> is the fact that issues surrounding race, culture and their attendant problems are often more urgent concerns than social class. Too many liberal community organizers have emphasized class issues at the expense of racism and cultural chauvinism, relegating them to 'logical' extensions of the political and economic structure. Much of the neo-Marxist literature has treated race from a reductive, negative posture. (Rivera & Erlich, 1992, p. 6)

In addition conservative thinkers have overemphasized uniqueness of particular communities and have separated those who can and those who cannot "make it" in mainstream society. Rivera and Erlich stress culture as their central organizing principle, citing it as: "a collection of behaviors and beliefs that constitute 'standards for deciding what is, standards for deciding what can be, standards for deciding how one feels about it, standards for deciding what to do about it, and standards for deciding how to go about doing it' " (p. 9). For all communities of color in America, factors of importance are: (1) the racial, ethnic, and cultural uniqueness of people; (2) the implications of these unique qualities within their group and in the larger society; and (3) "the process of empowerment and the development of critical consciousness" (p. 11). The book proceeds to specific chapters covering the following groups: Native Americans, Chicanos, African-Americans, Puerto Ricans, Chinese Americans, Japanese Americans, Central American Immigrants, Southeast Asians, and chapters on a feminist perspective, community development and restoration; and the 1990s.

From examination of the ten chapters in their book dealing with specific groups, Rivera and Erlich build a "Model in Progress" based on the following components (pp. 14-20):

1. Similar cultural and racial identification.
2. Familiarity with customs and traditions, etc.
3. Intimate knowledge of language and sub-group slang.
4. Knowledge of leadership styles and development.
5. An analytical framework for political and economic analysis.
6. Knowledge of past organizing strategies–strengths and limitations.
7. Skills in conscientization and empowerment.
8. Skills in assessing community psychology.
9. Knowledge of organizational behavior.
10. Skills in evaluative and participatory research.
11. Skills in program planning, development and administration.
12. An awareness of self and personal strengths and limitations.

The importance of adding this base of knowledge, areas of concern and skills for community practice cannot be underestimated as the nation moves into the twenty first century. The anti-racist model described by Popple (this volume) offers useful guides for strengthening community practice in diverse communities and building an anti-racist society. New understandings of diversity and oppression argue eloquently for commitment to social and economic empowerment for communities of color and marginalized groups, for stronger multi-cultural consciousness and a commitment to equality and opportunity for all members of society.

Rothman Redux, 1995

After presenting an early draft at the ACOSA Symposium in 1994, Jack Rothman published a major revision of his classic three models in the first two chapters of the Fifth Edition of *Strategies of Community Intervention: Macro Practice* (Rothman et al., 1995). Most of that new work is reprinted here in this volume and responded to in articles by Hyde and Jeffries. In this reworking of his earlier material, Rothman moves from the comparison of selected practice variable in relation to locality development, social planning and social action, to a treatment of the basic three models, first as ideal-types and then as overlapping interventions with mid-points of mixed models: action/planning, development/action, and planning/development. A major part of the article describes types of organizations that fit the three major and three mixed models and the points between to define and illustrate a new "paradigm of community intervention" which presents examples of organizational types for each mode of intervention and each mixed form. The typology proceeds with examples of horizontally and vertically linked organizations, examples of concentrated and dispersed decision-making to illustrate citizen participation levels, and an example of goal and means analysis using "radical" and "normative" goals and "radical" and "normative" tactics to illustrate ways that the typology can be applied. This expanded and more specified typology is an exciting and useful means of analyzing community practice approaches. Rothman expresses the hope that the revision will spur more research on change processes and methods of intervention. This new paradigm asserts once again the value of typologies and analysis of models to assess community situations and plan appropriate interventions.

Eight Current Models of Community Practice: Weil and Gamble, 1995

During the early 1990s Weil and Gamble engaged in a broad-based survey of the literature and conducted research on existing models of community practice as part of curriculum development and writing projects in areas of citizen participation, community practice, and sustainable community development. The research process and the subsequent trial by fire of testing out ideas with classes and practitioners over a several year period resulted in development of a framework of eight basic models of community practice. The eight model typology was determined on the basis of multiple, thriving examples of each model extant in the mid-1990s, the connection of these models to earlier historical models, and the expectation that these eight models will persist over time.

A detailed description of these eight models was published in the 19th Edition of the *Encyclopedia of Social Work* as "Community Practice Models" (Weil & Gamble, 1995). This typology provides a framework of eight functionally specified models of community practice which have discrete and specialized purposes as illustrated in the distinctive desired outcomes of the models: (1) Neighborhood and Community Organizing; (2) Organizing Functional Communities;

(3) Community Social and Economic Development; (4) Social Planning; (5) Program Development and Community Liaison; (6) Political and Social Action; (7) Coalitions; and (8) Social Movements. The models are described in terms of the following comparative characteristics: desired outcome; system targeted for change, primary constituency; scope of concern; and social work roles, as illustrated in Table 1.

There is no assumption that these models are mutually exclusive. They may exist as mixed models such as Rothman's (1995) depiction of mixed aspects (e.g., of social action and planning). They may be sequentially used within an organization or emerge sequentially as an organization or group changes or expands its foci–for example, a progression from organizing for neighborhood needs to development of community or group controlled services as described by Grosser and Mondros (1995) in political action approaches and by Gottlieb (1980), Weil (1986), Bricker-Jenkins and Hooyman (1986), Perlmutter (1994), and Hyde (1995) in the development of feminist alternative services for women. These eight models also have some overlap in conceptual components and in roles that workers will take. However, each model is analytically discrete, often discrete in practice, and represents a specific, coherent, and clear approach to community practice. It is hoped that these eight models are useful in teaching by providing a typology that can be used in assessment and strategy selection, in evaluation of interventions by practitioners, and in comparative research.

This framework is distinct from Rothman's original (1976) and revised model typologies (this volume) in several ways and different from the five model presentation of Taylor and Roberts (1985). This framework clearly specifies distinctions between and among (a) organizing in neighborhoods and geographic communities, (b) organizing in functional communities, and (c) community social and economic development. Rothman has never fully treated the distinctions between local geographic organizing and the complexity of organizing functional communities which can occur at local, regional, state, national or international levels.

In addition, as is evident in the historical literature there have been considerable distinctions between the enabling/empowering/conscientization focus of social development as written about by Ross (1955, 1958), Lappin (1985), and Reisch and Wenocur (1986),

TABLE 1. Current Models of Community Practice for Social Work

	Models							
Comparative Characteristics	Neighborhood and Community Organizing	Organizing Functional Communities	Community Social and Economic Development	Social Planning	Program Development and Community Liaison	Political and Social Action	Coalitions	Social Movements
Desired outcome	Develop capacity of members to organize; change the impact of citywide planning and external development	Action for social justice focused on advocacy and on changing behaviors and attitudes; may also provide service	Initiate development plans from a grassroots perspective; prepare citizens to make use of social and economic investments	Citywide or regional proposals for action by elected body or human services planning councils	Expansion or redirection of agency program to improve community service effectiveness; organize new service	Action for social justice focused on changing policy or policy makers	Build a multiorganizational power base large enough to influence program direction or draw down resources	Action for social justice that provides a new paradigm for a particular population group or issue
System targeted or change	Municipal government; external developers; community members	General public; government institutions	Banks; foundations; external developers; community citizens	Perspectives of community leaders; perspectives of human services leaders	Funders of agency programs; beneficiaries of agency services	Voting public; elected officials; inactive/ potential participants	Elected officials; foundations; government institutions	General public: political systems
Primary constituency	Residents of neighborhood, parish, or rural county	Like-minded people in a community, region, nation, or across the globe	Low-income, marginalized, or oppressed population groups in a city or region	Elected officials; social agencies and interagency organizations	Agency board or administrators; community representatives	Citizens in a particular political jurisdiction	Organizations that have a stake in the particular issue	Leaders and organizations able to create new visions and images

TABLE 1 (continued)

	Models							
Comparative Characteristics	Neighborhood and Community Organizing	Organizing Functional Communities	Community Social and Economic Development	Social Planning	Program Development and Community Liaison	Political and Social Action	Coalitions	Social Movements
Scope of concern	Quality of life in the geographic area	Advocacy for particular issue or population	Income, resource, and social support development; improved basic education and leadership skills	Integration of social needs into geographic planning in public arena; human services network coordination	Service development for a specific population	Building political power; institutional change	Specified issue related to social need or concern	Social justice within society
Social work roles	Organizer Teacher Coach Facilitator	Organizer Advocate Writer/ communicator Facilitator	Negotiator Promoter Teacher Planner Manager	Researcher Proposal writer Communicator Manager	Spokesperson Planner Manager Proposal writer	Advocate Organizer Researcher Candidate	Mediator Negotiator Spokesperson	Advocate Facilitator

Weil, M. & Gamble, D. (1995) "Community Practice Models," *Encyclopedia of Social Work*, 19th Edition, pp. 577-594 and the more technical focus of many economic development efforts as described by Rubin and Rubin (1992) and Twelvetrees (1989). The evident need now is to combine social and economic development so that people, communities, and the planet are sustainable (Estes, 1993; Hoff, 1994; Midgeley, 1995). In this framework, therefore, social and economic development are explicitly combined.

The eight model framework, in contrast to Rothman's conceptualization, articulates three specific models focused on social change: (1) political and social action, (2) coalitions, and (3) social movements. Rothman's original conception and the current revision do not seem to have a logical place for coalitions, and they are indeed a growing part of community practice in areas related to health, mental health, and the environment. The complexity of practice with coalitions reframes some of the intergroup focus of the 1940s and '50s, and the methods of practice with coalitions and the tensions in their unity and diversity are more clearly specified in works by Mizrahi and Rosenthal (1993), and Roberts DeGennaro (1987, 1986). Social movements clearly are a major aspect of community practice which can change major life conditions and promote social justice. From abolition to the labor movement to civil rights, welfare rights, the disability movement, the women's movement, and environmental movements, social workers have been and are frequently engaged as members, facilitators, and advocates. In their scope, social movements are distinct from other social action and are therefore treated in this typology as a separate model.

The Weil and Gamble framework carries forward from Rothman (1976) and Taylor and Roberts (1985) a specified model of social planning; however, it also recognizes the discreteness of the program development model articulated by Kurzman (1985), which Rothman's work has not given attention, and combines it with the community liaison model as formulated by Taylor (1985). Both program development and community liaison functions were seen as historically validated in the '40s and '50s and as having growing importance currently. However, examination of recent case studies and practice examples indicated that these two aspects of community work are and should be carried out together under the rubric of one model. With the ever increasing emphasis on empowerment-focused programs, it is important that program development not be carried out without strong consumer or potential consumer involvement and that liaison to community groups most frequently takes place in the context of program planning, expansion or change or increasingly in enlarged community-based accountability and governance functions.

Given the historical focus of this article, only the basic purpose and desired outcomes of the eight models can be discussed. A detailed analysis of each model with current practice examples is provided in the article "Community Practice Models" in the 19th Edition of the *Encyclopedia of Social Work* (Weil & Gamble, 1995). For this discussion only the essential purpose and desired outcomes of the models will be emphasized.

Neighborhood and Community Organizing is a practice model designed to assist residents of a local area to organize and work together to build power and improve the quality of life in their geographic area. Its purpose is to initiate positive change in the social, physical and economic environment of the given area. The primary process is organizing–to identify issues, set goals, determine needed change strategies, and to implement and evaluate those strategies. Organizing also focuses on conscientization and capacity building to assist residents in developing skills needed to achieve their goals. There is an approximately equal focus on capacity building and task accomplishment.

Workers are most often engaged in helping to develop democratic functional leadership in which group members are able to build on and rely on each others' skills, use participatory democratic decision-making processes to set goals, and develop assessment, problem analysis, research, and action strategies to achieve their goals. Depending on the identified problems and desired goals, strategies may be cooperative, collaborative or adversarial. Goals may be political, social, environmental, or economic in focus and often combine these areas. Increasingly local organizing efforts are evolving into planning, creation, implementation and evaluation of projects, programs or services designed "from the grassroots up" with an ongoing investment in local control.

The knowledge base for this model derives from the rich community organizing practice literature, from sociology and community theory, from ideological analyses of social problems, and from theories related to strategies of conflict, collaboration and cooperation. Local community organizing can and does occur in high population density urban neighborhoods, in exurban areas and in rural communities. The desired outcome (major goal) of this model of practice is to combine the capacity building, and leadership development processes with development of skills in organizing, problem analysis, strategy selection, implementation and evaluation in order to achieve the goals set by the community group. In many instances organizing is focused on achieving desired change by influencing municipal government, by changing priorities for development, by building a strong constituency in the area to protect its people and resources, and to assist in change and development that is grounded in local goal setting and decision-making. A major result of organizing should be changes in power relations so that the group and the community have greater influence on decisions that affect their lives and neighborhoods. The central purpose then of this model is to develop the capacity of members to organize effectively, develop appropriate strategies, and build power and influence to achieve desired goals in their social, political, economic, and physical environment.

Organizing Functional Communities. This practice model focuses on organizing communities of interest–that is, forming groups of people into organizations committed to positive change in a specific area of concern. Its primary purpose is to effect social change regarding the special concern through enabling and empowering members to advocate effectively for their issues. Organizing is again the primary process. Workers will assist those who have targeted an issue in identifying and recruiting others of like mind to build an organization commited to change for a particular issue or population. Educating and advocating are major strategies. The constituency will be people of like mind and the scope can be from local to global (local Associations of Retarded Citizens to Amnesty International). Often there is a process of conscientization for potential group/organization members followed by use of educational and advocacy strategies to influence the general public, the media, public institutions and governmental organizations. "The central purpose and desired outcome in organizing functional communities is action for social justice focused on advocacy and on changing policies, behaviors, and attitudes in relation to their chosen issue" (Weil & Gamble, 1995, p. 583). Functional communities are also increasingly developing services related to their concerns such as respite care for children with emotional and behavioral disorders. Staff may assist groups in research, policy analysis and policy approach development, lobbying, direct social action, education campaigns and service development. These tasks require skills in facilitation, member recruitment, organizing and advocacy and often advanced skills in communications, information processing, and materials development. The geographic dispersion of members heightens the importance of use of technology in internal as well as external communications and education. Many functional communities conduct research on their issues and organize education and advocacy campaigns around their findings. The central function of functional community organizations is the achievement of social justice in their specified area through changing policies and social behaviors.

Community Social and Economic Development. This new typology merges social and economic development, recognizing that in low-income, oppressed, or isolated communities creation of stronger and more sustainable institutions and resources requires attention and success in both areas (NCCED, 1991). This model also increasingly incorporates principles and practices of sustainable development for both populations and environmental resources. Its central purpose is to build capacity among people to plan and initiate their own projects to improve social conditions, and build economic resources and opportunities in keeping with the culture of the community and appropriate to its natural environment. Its functions combine conscientization, skills development in decision-making and planning processes and in development of specific task and technical skills for particular projects. Community members themselves are the major system targeted for change with concomitant focus on effecting changes in and influencing the policies and practices of government agents, external developers, or funding sources such as foundations. Lappin (1985) stresses the enabling role in community development; however, the successful transformation of community and achievement of goals such as developing needed low income housing or development of cooperative economic ventures, or micro enterprise support through peer lending groups are equally important. Workers may be involved in work with developing groups, helping to build cohesion, serving as a coach/educator for particular skills such as planning and negotiation, and may train residents for or initially carry responsibilities for planning and managing projects. Development projects take place in communities (rural, urban and regional) throughout the world. Internationally as well as in the U.S., increasing focus has been given to empowerment strategies and developing local control of projects and resources. The movement for sustainable development and opposition to environmental racism (and promotion of environmental justice) has evolved in large part in response to major failures in externally controlled or "prepackaged development projects." The success of community development rests in the commitment and ownership of the local population and the development of appropriate and sustainable technology for economic enterprises. The central purpose of development that is grounded in social justice is the development of people–their capacities and skills–so that they can initiate and maintain grassroots plans and projects, improve their social and economic conditions, and support and sustain their home environment and its resources. This type of development can be viewed as community transformation.

Social Planning has sometimes been defined or described extremely broadly to cover almost all aspects of community practice and sometimes more narrowly to embrace only those efforts by governmental or coordinating councils that are devoted to providing the best possible information (both quantity and quality) to inform decisions and to increase "the use of rational techniques in the decision-making process itself" (Gummer, 1995). In this typology the definition takes more of a middle ground. Social planning surely includes the classic rational planning models grounded in specialized expertise and research and data utilization; and it certainly needs to include an emphasis on rational decision-making (Kahn, 1969; Brager & Specht, 1969; Gummer, 1995). It is increasingly common to find public and nonprofit partnership or broader community collaborative efforts engaging in social planning for human services. Lauffer's 1981 definition fits well with the typology developed by Weil and Gamble: "Social Planning refers to the development, expansion, and coordination of social services and social policies" that is a model of practice relying on rational problem-solving that can occur in organizations ranging in scale from local to national or international focus (Lauffer, 1981, p. 583).

Social planning can focus primarily on coordinating human services or engage in planning that more broadly integrates social and economic concerns. Major shifts in social policy directions have taken place and are continuing through the work of Congress. While many of these shifts are punishing of the poor, of oppressed communities, and increasingly of the working and lower middle class, there may well be opportunities for planners at state and county levels (in both governmental and nonprofit sectors) to focus planning on more adaptive and relevant responses to local or state needs. The majority of "formal" social planning has often occurred in the deliberations on citywide or regional proposals that are acted upon by elected bodies or by human service planning councils–with little input from those most affected by proposed policy and practice changes. Very often elected officials and interagency organizations may be the primary participants and or constituencies represented in more formal social planning processes. However, if the scope of concern cited by Weil and Gamble, "integration of social needs into geographic planning in the public arena," and human services network collaboration is taken seriously, the broader reaches of social planning must be taken in (1995).

Tensions within "expert" oriented models were duly noted by Brager and Specht in the 1960s and '70s, and more recently, critical theory and feminist critiques of social processes and problems have emphasized the importance of multiple voices and perspectives as critical for good planning. While local groups in rural areas, for example, may not have all the language of technical planners, they will often know much more realistically what their land and environment and population can bear and support (Sager, 1996, personal communication). For example, Noponen has developed a participatory monitoring and evaluation tool that is being piloted with grassroots micro-lending programs in India. Pictorial diaries are used so that literacy is not needed and the system is built on participatory research and problem solving. Experts have a great deal to learn from local communities, and their positions are not at all necessarily "nonrational." Clearly at both local and international development levels social planning that was not grounded in local knowledge and wisdom about land and peoples has produced massive failures. Advocacy planning was popular in the late '60s and '70s and often brought useful technical skills to local groups to assist them in planning for housing and economic development or for rural community regeneration. Serious planning takes place in Community Development Corporations and in multi-system collaborations in human services. This combination that Rothman (1995) describes as Development/Planning is a critical approach if democracy is taken seriously and if sustainable social plans are to be developed and implemented. Workers engaged in social planning might be connected to official elected bodies or governmental bureaucracies, they might be employees of human service planning councils or they might work with local groups, national organizations, or coalitions–both rural and urban–on developing appropriate and responsive plans that incorporate planning and research for economic, environmental, and social resources. Lauffer notes major roles for planners at four levels: direct service agencies, service sectors, comprehensive local planning structure, and regional or intersectorial or intergovernmental planning structures (1978). At this point in time with the environmental risks evident near the turn of the century, the problems created in global structural adjustment strategies, and the emergence of the global economy, it is ever more important that planners at all levels learn to communicate and work productively with the people who live with the conditions on which planners are focused. Technical expertise is of great importance, but research methods and planning skills can be taught and caught by local groups as Gaventa's and others' work demonstrates (Gaventa, 1980). Planning is a process that is carried on in most community practice processes; where it is the dominant focus and model, it is important that social planning not maintain a kind of exclusive focus on expertise and that planners recognize the risks of making "rational" decisions that in fact represent the interests of powerful ingroups (or the current status quo). Planning needs to broaden into providing more effective and inclusive means of interchange of information and involvement in analysis, research, and decision making. Broader participation is likely to bring about better decisions and longer term societal benefits for more diverse groups.

The need to strengthen participation and to broaden skills in planning is one real tension facing the field at this point in time. Gummer (1995) provides careful analysis of other tensions citing (1) the increasingly politically punitive view of the poor, (2) the rapid increase in the for-profit sector in human services, and (3) the (survival focused) response to both these trends in the nonprofit sector to focus increasingly on fee for service, third party reimbursement and for-profit ventures. The central risk that he analyzes is the likelihood that this combination of factors will refocus the social service sector from the needs of the poor and most vulnerable to those most able to pay for services (Gummer, 1995). Citing Hirshfield's options of "exit, voice, or loyalty," Gummer notes that many social workers have exited (or been squeezed out of) planning roles in government and in community welfare systems; others have striven to give "voice" to the needs of the less and least advantaged, and some have opted for bureaucratic loyalty to organizations whose goals have shifted more to protectionism than to maintenance of mission. While the pressures of individualism, materialism and an almost exclusively bottom-line focus that Gummer notes are all too real, there are also countervailing values related to increasing local control of services, increasing focus on interagency and human service system collaboration, and increasing opportunities to develop and use local and state-level research and data to shed light and bring rationality to social planning and decision-making.

Program Development and Community Liaison. This model merges two approaches previously treated separately by Kurzman (1985) and Taylor (1985). Combining these models seems warranted because community liaison activities are an essential aspect of program development. The purpose and desired outcome of this model is the creation of a new service, or the expansion or redirection of an agency program to improve responsiveness to community needs. The community liaison function particularly specified the engagement of client, potential clients and community members in assessment of needs and articulation of service goals to assure appropriateness to the population. This model most often is used in agencies whose primary function is not community practice. The liaison responsibility becomes the major connection between the agency and the people it serves. Major emphasis is placed on increasing and making more effective the interaction between citizens, potential clients, and agency staff. These interactions can be strengthened by "the involvement of potential consumers and citizens in the needs assessment process, utilization of focus groups of potential consumers and/or related agency staff, development of advisory bodies and involvement of potential consumers and community leaders in policy making boards. As the program is designed and implemented, mechanisms for feedback to and from the community are valuable in keeping new programs on target" (Weil & Gamble, 1995, p. 587).

In a sense, by emphasizing the liaison function, the agency targets itself for change as well as potential clients. Planners or liaison staff will work with both agency boards, other agency representatives and community representatives in the program design process.

Service development for a particular population or geographic area comprises the scope of this model. "Roles likely to be taken on by the worker include planner, and proposal writer, spokesperson, mediator, and facilitator in the interaction process with constituent groups and external supporters. As the program becomes established, the worker will often take on roles of manager, monitor and evaluator to assure that the program stays on-track, meets its goals for service and change and remains responsive to the community and changing environment" (Weil & Gamble, 1995, p. 587). The significance of this model is its greatly increased emphasis on developing more mutual planning strategies with community members.

Political and Social Action. This model is patterned from practice reality and clearly draws on earlier articulation by Rothman (1979), Grosser and Mondros (1985), Reisch and Wenocur (1986), Rubin and Rubin (1992) and Hanna and Robinson (1994). The purpose of this model is to facilitate action for social justice focused on changing policy or policy makers or changing actions of corporations that disadvantage low-income groups. Strategies challenge inequalities that limit opportunities and involve direct confrontation of decision-makers who have ignored community needs. Social action efforts dispute unjust decisions, empower people through strengthening their belief in their own efficacy, and develop their skills to change unjust conditions (Rubin & Rubin, 1992; Staples, 1990). Rubin and Rubin note: "Social action campaigns document a problem, choose as a target those who can effect a solution, symbolize the issue, take pressureful actions and try to ensure the implementation of promised changes" (Rubin & Rubin, 1992, p. 245). The major goal is to shift the balance of power so that those who have been excluded in earlier decision making processes become "players" in future decisions. This goal is grounded in actions to strengthen participatory democracy and values for building social justice.

Through participation, members of the social/political change effort develop organizing and leadership skills. Capacity building may involve investigative research and use of findings to change plans or decisions. Social action groups are involved in educating their community or constituencies about their issue, recruiting members for a variety of roles, and taking direct action. "Members must be confident of their skills to plan actions and convinced of the legitimacy of their cause and tactics. Public elected and administrative officials are often targets for change in social and political action. Other targets of change may be major corporations or businesses that have been engaged in activities damaging to the community such as pollution of the environment or endangering the health and livelihood of the workers. Action groups also want to educate the public to understand their cause and the mobilization of public opinion can become a major part of an action campaign" (Weil & Gamble, 1995, pp. 587-588).

The primary constituency of a direct action group is citizens in a particular political jurisdiction, or citizens or workers committed to a particular cause. While there is great diversity in the causes that will be pursued through direct action, the scope of concern of all will be building political power and promoting institutional change toward greater social justice. Roles for social workers in political and social action will include advocate, educator, organizer and researcher. Internally the organizer will be engaged in capacity building, both in terms of internal group process and decision-making skills and in externally focused skills in direct action, public and media relations and investigative research. While the organizer may directly serve as an advocate in some instances, it is much more important that the organizer assist group members in becoming their own advocates. "Much of the organizer's work is in facilitative leadership and capacity building" (Weil & Gamble, 1995, p. 588).

"Grassroots organizing for political and social action requires not only skills in organizing, but increasingly requires skills in research, computer utilization, media and public relations as well as fundraising skills for long term projects which may grow out of the action process. Grosser and Mondros (1985) note that social action groups may decide to develop their own programs and services so that models will be appropriate and empowering. When such programs are implemented, groups must also master fundraising, communication, and management skills needed for nonprofit administration" (Weil & Gamble, 1995, p. 588).

Coalitions. Social Change Coalitions are defined by Mizrahi and Rosenthal as "a group of diverse organizational representatives who join forces to influence external institutions on one or more issues affecting their constituencies while maintaining their own autonomy" (1993, p. 14). Coalitions generally will have a time-limited life span typically filled with dynamic tensions resulting from the simultaneous demands on organizational representatives to remain autonomous as representatives of their "home" organizations while at the same time building an amalgamated organization by defining and acting on the shared interests of the various member organizations.

The purpose of coalitions is most often to build a multiorganizational power base large enough to influence social program direction and/or effectively demand resources for the purpose of responding to the common interests of the coalition. Elected officials and government organizations are most often targets for change in policies and resource allocation.

Generally, because coalition building requires an enormous time commitment, only organizations that have a considerable stake in a particular issue will participate in coalitions, because they require a great time commitment to have likelihood of success. The scope of concern for social change coalitions is building political power and promoting institutional change on the specific issue or issues which member groups can agree to support. In order to stay together, coalitions develop complex exchange relations and find ways to balance their commitment to the issues that hold them together with the individual agendas and perspectives of member groups (Roberts-DeGennaro, 1986, 1987). "Social workers are likely to be leaders and spokespersons in professional or human service coalitions. To build and maintain the coalition, mediation and negotiation skills are often critical to balance tensions and maintain the coalition's focus" (Weil & Gamble, 1995, p. 589).

Social Movements are a model of community practice that extends beyond social work as a profession. Many social workers are and have been engaged in social change movements whose purpose is action for social justice. When social movements are successful they provide a new paradigm for a particular population, group or issue–that is, they may define and extend civil rights or foster protection rather than exploitation of the environment. As a profession social work typically has not been the prime mover in social movements, but many members will be involved and the nature of practice is influenced by current social movements. "Sometimes progress toward a just and caring society is assisted by social movements as in the case of the Civil Rights Movement and at other times it may be impeded, as in the case of the movements spawned as the result of homophobia. Social workers, in keeping with the values of the profession will be allied with social movements that support democracy, individual dignity, the rights of minorities, the needs of the poor, sustainable development, and activities that support broad goals of human development and liberation" (Weil & Gamble, 1995, p. 589).

The systems targeted for change by social movements generally are the public, the media, and political systems. "In the US, the Civil Rights Movement is perhaps the best known and most far-reaching recent example of a social movement. Over time its leaders balanced coalitions and managed social change in policies, laws, organizations, institutions, and attitudes and behaviors. In many ways the Civil Rights movement fathered civil and social rights activities in La Raza, the Women's Movement and the later Disabilities Rights Movement. In each of these movements, new paradigms about these groups emerged with the success of the movement. Both legislation and attitudes have begun to focus more on abilities than disabilities; women increasingly exercise equal rights and move into leadership positions; and while racism and prejudice have not disappeared, Latinos, African Americans, and Native Americans have established civil rights and continue to work towards social and economic equality. Many social workers have been involved in each of these movements as volunteers and as organizational staff. Their roles often were those of advocate and facilitator" (Weil & Gamble, 1995, p. 589). As a social movement succeeds, the ideals that it has advanced are accepted as new, legitimized political and social norms.

CONCLUSIONS: OVERARCHING FRAMEWORK FOR COMMUNITY PRACTICE

The models presented here illustrate the current range and major modes of community practice. As Rothman (1979) has noted, actual practice may combine aspects of various models and may be phased sequentially over time as a neighborhood organization grows into intensive work in economic or social development, or a community of interest builds a needed alternative service system. Local groups increasingly see their connections to global issues and actions. Models can guide practice, but they are not static rubrics. Practice will continue to change in response to local and international issues and internal and external environmental influences.

Each of the eight models presented has a discrete primary purpose and function and mirrors the realities of current practice. They also are long lived enough over the period from the 1920s until now (though in various incarnations adapted to the prevailing social and economic conditions and the stage of development of the literature and the profession) that they can reasonably be expected to continue as viable models. In combination, these models provide a framework, that is, a structure or design to provide the conceptual support, for assessment, analysis and evaluation of current situations in relation to the specified, discretely identified "ideal types" that provide models or patterns through which to analyze, plan, and evaluate interventions. This framework is a useful teaching tool and is useful in community situations to assess what approach is called for or most appropriate. Analysis of the scope of concern, primary constituency, system targeted for change and, most critically, the desired outcome, can assist in selection of most appropriate strategies for intervention. Finally analysis of the role set taken on by practitioners in each model can be useful as a teaching tool in educational programs and is as well useful in clarifying roles for practitioners.

Heuristically, a model should be simple enough to be understandable and teachable; it should take account of theoretical and practice complexities; it should help to make complex situations more understandable–by using the abstraction or "ideal type" of the model to see if it is useful in interpreting and elaborating current situations. If so then the framework becomes a means to specify action plans by analysis of the comparative characteristics as a backdrop to selection of appropriate strategy–and a test to see that selected strategies are appropriate to the desired outcome or major purpose of the model.

This set of models also has utility in that it encompasses the range (from neighborhood organizing to mass social movements) and the scope (from local to global concerns) of community practice. These models are *functional* in that they "are designed for or adapted to a particular need or activity" (*American Heritage Dictionary*, 1980). The basic functions embodied by this eight model framework combine to embody the four overarching processes of community practice: organizing, planning, development and social change for social justice (Weil, 1994). *Process* denotes "a series of actions, changes, or functions that bring about an end or result" as well as movement and progression over time (*AH*, 1980). The functional focus and the process needed to implement a model are critical elements in achieving the goal or purpose of a particular model (as it is used to assess, analyze, and evaluate a particular situation). Purpose encompasses the intention, goals, and desired outcomes of a model. These purposes and major functions define community practice, clarify its domain, and illustrate its great diversity. The following chart presents the eight models organized by their overarching process and purpose:

CHART 1. Overarching Processes and Purposes of Eight Current Models of Community Practice

Development:

Social and Economic Development–sustainable development at neighborhood, local community, regional, national, international and global levels

Organizing:

Neighborhood and Community Organizing;
Organizing Functional Communities.

Planning:

Program Development and Community Liaison;
Social Planning–at all levels.

Change:

Political and Social Action;
Coalitions; and
Social Movements.

This simplified chart structure may assist is using the eight models as an analytic and teaching tool.

NOTES

1. The literature since 1945 is rich and varied and deserves a careful history. Jack Rothman has a project in progress to present that history including reflections by major writers on their own work and directions in community practice.
2. My apology to the authors whose work deserves to be discussed in its contribution to the thinking and work of the time!

REFERENCES

Adams, F. with Horton, M. (1975). Unearthing seeds of fire: The idea of highlander. Winston-Salem, NC: Blair.

Addams, J. (1960). *A centennial reader.* NY: The MacMillian Co.

Addams, J. (1895). "The settlement as a factor in the labor movement" in *Hull-House maps and papers, by residents of Hull-House, a social settlement, a presentation of nationalities and wages in a congested district of Chicago, together with comments and essays on problems growing out of the social conditions*. New York: Crowell.

Addams, J. (1910) *Twenty years at Hull-House.* New York: MacMillan.

Addams, J. (1930). *The second twenty years at Hull-House.* New York: MacMillan.

Addams, J. (1920). *Democracy and social ethics.* New York: MacMillian.

Alinsky, S. (1971). *Rules for radicals.* New York: Random House.

Asian American Mental Health Training Center (1981). *Bridging cultures: social work with Southeast Asian Refugees.* Los Angeles: AAMHTC & Special Services for Groups.

Austin, M. J., & Betten, N. (1990). Rural organizing and the agricultural extension service. In Betten, N. & Austin M. J. (Eds.) *The roots of community organizing, 1917-1939.* Philadelphia: Temple University Press, pp. 94-105.

Bennis, W. G., Benne, Kenneth D., & Chin. (1961). *The planning of change.* New York: Holt, Rinehart and Winston.

Betten, N. & Austin M. J. (Eds.) (1990). *The roots of community organizing, 1917-1939.* Philadelphia: Temple University Press.

Betten, N. & Austin M. J. (1990). The conflict approach to community organizing: Saul Alinsky and the CIO. In Betten, N. & Austin M.J. (Eds.) *The roots of community organizing, 1917-1939.* Philadelphia: Temple University Press, pp. 152-161.

Biddle, W. W. & Biddle, L. J. (1965). *The community development process.* New York: Holt, Rinehart and Winston.

Blakely, E. J. (1979). *Community development research: Concepts, issues and strategies.* New York: Human Sciences Press.

Blakely, E. J. (1989). *Planning local economic development: Theory and practice.* Newbury Park, CA: Sage.

Bobo, K., Kendall, J., & Max, S. (1991). *Organizing for social change: A manual for activists in the 1990's.* Washington, DC: Seven Locks Press.

Bradshaw, C., Soifer, S. & Gutierrez, L. (1994). Toward a hybrid model for effective organizing in communities of color. *Journal of Community Practice,* 1(1), pp. 25-41.

Brager, G., & Specht, H. (1973). *Community organizing.* New York: Columbia University Press.

Branch, T. (1988) *Parting the waters: America in the King years, 1954-63.* New York: Simon & Schuster.

Brandwein, R. A. (1981). Toward androgyny in community and organizational practice. In A. Weick & S. T. Vandiver (Eds.), *Women, power & change* (pp. 158-170). Washington, DC: NASW.

Bricker-Jenkins, M. & Hooyman, N. (1986). A feminist world view: Ideological themes from the feminist movement. In M. Bricker-Jenkins & N. Hooyman (Eds.), *Not for women only: Social work practice for a feminist future* (pp. 7-21). Washington, DC: NASW.

Carlton-LaNey, I. (June 1994). The career of Birdye Henrietta Haynes, a pioneer settlement house worker. *Social Service Review, 68* (2), pp. 254-273.

Carlton-LaNey, I. & Burwell, Y. (1996). Introduction to Special Issue. *Journal of Community Practice, 2* (4).

Carter, G. W. (1959). "Practice theory in community organization," in Lurie, H. L. (Ed.) (1959). *The Community organization method in social work education, Volume IV*, a project report of the curriculum study, Werner W. Boehm, Director & Coordinator. New York: Council on Social Work Education.

Chavis, David M., Florin, P. & Felix, M. R. J. (1993). Nurturing grassroots initiatives for community development: The role of enabling systems. In Terry Mizrahi & John D. Morrison (Eds.). *Community organization and social administration*. NY: The Haworth Press, Inc., pp. 41-67.

Christenson, J. A. & Robinson, J.W. Jr. (1989). *Community development in perspective*. Ames, IA: Iowa State University Press.

Cordoba, C. (1992). Organizing in Central American immigrant communities in the United States. In Rivera, F. & Erlich, J. (Eds.) *Community organizing in a diverse society*. Boston: Allyn and Bacon, pp. 181-200.

Cox, F. M., Erlich, J. L., Rothman, J., & Tropman. (1970). *Strategies of community organization.* Itasca, IL: Peacock.

Cox, F. M., Erlich, J. L., Rothman, J., & Tropman, J. E. (Eds.) (1984). *Tactics and techniques of community practice*, Second Edition. Itasca IL: Peacock.

Cox, F., Erlich, J. L., Rothman, J. and Tropman, J. E. (eds.) (1987). *Strategies of community organization*, Fourth Edition. Itasca IL: F.E. Peacock.

Dahl, Robert. (1985). *A Preface to economic democracy.* Berkeley and Los Angeles: University of California Press, pp. 162-63.

Dahl, Robert. (1989). *Democracy and its critics.* New Haven: Yale University Press.

Daley, J. M. & Wong, P. (1994). Community development with emerging ethnic communities. *Journal of Community Practice*, 1(1), pp. 9-24.

Deegan, M. J. (1990). *Jane Addams and the men of the Chicago School, 1892-1918.* New Brunswick: Transaction Books.

Duncan, C. M. (1992). *Rural poverty in America.* New York: Auburn House.

Dunham, A. (1959). *Community welfare organization: Principles and practice.* New York: Thomas Y. Crowell Co.

Dunham, A. (1940). The literature of community organization, in *Proceedings of the National Conference of Social Work.* New York: Columbia University Press.

Ecklein, J. L., & Lauffer, A. A. (1972). *Community organizers and social planners*. New York: John Wiley & Sons and CSWE.

Edwards, R. L. (Ed.) (1995). *Encyclopedia of social work, Nineteenth Edition.* Washington, DC: NASW.

Edwards, E. D. & Egbert-Edwards, M. (1992). Native American community development, in Rivera, F. & Erlich, J. (Eds.), *Community organizing in a diverse society.* Boston: Allyn and Bacon. pp. 27-48.

Estes, R. J. (1993). Toward sustainable development: From theory to praxis. *Social Development Issues*, 15(3), pp. 1-29

Fisher, R. (1984). *Let the people decide: Neighborhood organizing in America.* Boston: Twayne.

Foner, P. S. (Ed.) (1970). *W.E.B. DuBois speaks: Speeches and addresses 1890-1919.* New York: Pathfinder Press.

Franklin, J. H. (1965). The two worlds of race: A historical view, *Daedalus* 94 (4), pp. 899-920.

Freire, P. (1981). *Pedagogy of the oppressed.* New York: Continuum Press.

Garvin, C. D. & Cox, F. M. (1995) A history of community organizing since the Civil War with special reference to oppressed communities, Chapter 2 in Rothman, J., Erlich, J. L., & Tropman, J. E. (Eds.), *Strategies of community intervention, Fifth Edition.* Itasca, IL: Peacock, pp. 64-99.

Gaventa, John. (1980). *Power and powerlessness: Quiescence and rebellion in an Appalachian valley.* Champaign-Urbana, IL: University of Illinois Press.

Gottlieb, N. (Ed.). (1980). *Alternative social services for women.* New York: Columbia University Press.

Grosser, C. F. & Mondros, J. (1985). Pluralism and participation: The political action approach, in Taylor and Roberts (Eds.), *Theory and practice of community social work.* New York: Columbia University Press. pp. 154-178.

Gummer, B. (1995). Social planing in Edwards, R. L. (Ed.) *Encyclopedia of social work, Nineteenth Edition.* Washington, DC: NASW, pp. 2180-2186.

Gurin, A. (1959). Community organization methods and skills in the programs of national agencies," in Lurie, H. L. (Ed.) (1959), *The community organization method in social work education, Volume IV,* A project report of the curriculum study, Werner W. Boehm, Director & Coordinator. New York: Council on Social Work Education.

Gurin, A. & Jones, W. (1970). *Community organizing and social planning.* New York: CSWE and John Wiley & Sons.

Gurteen, S. H. (November 1894). "Beginning of charity organization in America," *Lend a Hand*, Vol. 13, pp. 355-361.

Gurteen, S. H. (1882). *Handbook of charity organization.* Buffalo, NY (no publisher listed).

Gutierrez, L. M. & Lewis, E. A. (1994). Community organizing with women of color: A feminist approach. *Journal of Community Practice*, Vol. 1 (2) pp. 23-44.

Hall, Bob. (ed.). (1988). *Environmental politics: Lessons from the grassroots.* Durham, NC: Institute for Southern Studies.

Hanna, M. & Robinson, B. (1994). *Strategies for community empowerment.* Lewiston, NY: Edwin Melton Press.

Hart, J. K. (1920). *Community organization.* New York: MacMillan Company.

Harrington, M. (1962). *The Other America: Poverty in the United States.* New York: MacMillan.

Hoff, M. D. (1994). Environmental foundations of social welfare: Theoretical resources, in M. D. Hoff & J. G. McNutt (Eds.), *The global environmental crisis: Implications for social welfare and social work.* Brookfield, USA: Avebury. pp. 12-35.

Hooyman, N. R. & Bricker Jenkins, M. (1985). *Not for women only: Models of feminist practice.* Washington, DC: NASW.

Horton, M., with Kohl, J. & Kohl, H. (1990). *The long haul: An autobiography.* New York: Doubleday.

Hull-House Maps and Papers, by Residents of Hull-House, A Social Settlement, A Presentation of Nationalities and Wages in a Congested District of Chicago, Together With Comments and Essays on Problems Growing Out of the Social Conditions. (1895). New York: Crowell.

Hyde, C. (1986). Experience of women activists: Implications for community organizing theory. *Sociology & Social Welfare*, 13, pp. 545-562.

Johnson, A. (1959). Community organization method and skills in social casework practice, in H. L. Lurie (Ed.), *The community organization method in social work education*, Volume IV of the Project Report of the Social Work Curriculum Study. Washington, DC: CSWE, pp. 148-161.

Kahn, A. J. (1969). *Theory and practice of social planning.* New York: Russell Sage Foundation.

Kahn, S. (1982). *Organizing: A guide for grassroots leaders.* New York: McGraw-Hill.

Kettner, P., Daley, J. M. & Nichols, A. W. (1985). *Initiating change in organizations and communities: A macro practice model.* Monterey, CA: Brooks/Cole.

Kramer, R. M. & Specht, H. (Eds.) *Readings in community organization practice, Second Edition.* Englewood Cliffs, NJ: Prentice Hall.

Kurzman, P. (1985). Program development and service coordination as components of community practice, in Taylor and Roberts (Eds.), *Theory and practice of community social work.* New York: Columbia University Press. pp. 95-124.

Lane, R. P. (1939). The field of community organization–report of discussions. *The proceedings of the National Conference of Social Work: Selected papers from Sixty-sixth Annual Conference, Buffalo, New York June 18-24, 1939, Vol. 66.* Howard R. Knight, Ed. New York: Columbia University Press, pp. 495-511.

Lappin, B. (1985). Community development: Beginnings in social work enabling, in Taylor and Roberts (Eds.), *Theory and practice of community social work.* New York: Columbia University Press. pp. 59-94.

Lasch, C. (Ed.) (1965). Introduction to *The social thought of Jane Addams.* Indianapolis: Bobbs-Merrill.

Lauffer, A. (1981). The practice of social planning, in N. Gilbert & H. Specht (Eds.), *Handbook of the social services*, pp. 588-597. Englewood Cliffs, NJ: Prentice Hall.

Lauffer, A. (1978). *Social Planning at the community level.* Englewood Cliffs, NJ: Prentice Hall.

Lee, I. (1992). The Chinese-Americans community organizing strategies and tactics, in Rivera, F. G. & Erlich, J. L. (Eds.), *Community organizing in a diverse society.* Boston: Allyn and Bacon. pp. 133-158.

Lindeman, E. C. (1949). Democracy and social work, in *Proceedings National Conference of Social Work, 1948*. New York: Columbia University Press.

Lindeman, E. C. (1921). *The community: An introduction to the study of community leadership and organization*. New York: Association Press.

Lippitt, R., Watson J. & Westley, B. (1958). *The dynamics of planned change: A comparative study of principles and techniques*. New York: Harcourt, Brace & World.

Lord, R. (1939). *The agrarian revival.* American Association for Adult Education. New York: George Grady Press.

Lurie, H. L. (Ed.) (1959). *The community organization method in social work education, Volume IV,* A Project Report of the Curriculum Study, Werner W. Boehm, Director & Coordinator. New York: Council on Social Work Education.

Lurie, H. L. (Ed.) (1965). *Encyclopedia of social work. Fifteenth Issue*. New York: NASW.

McClenahan, B. A. (1925). *Organizing the community: A review of practical principles*. New York: Century Company.

McMillen, W. (1945). *Community organization for social welfare*. Chicago: University of Chicago Press.

Midgley. J. (1995). *Social development: The development perspective in social welfare*. Thousand Oaks, CA: SAGE.

Minahan, A. (Ed.) (1987). *Encyclopedia of social work: Eighteenth Edition*. Silver Spring MD: NASW.

Morris, R. (Ed.) (1971). *Encyclopedia of social work, Sixteenth Issue*. Washington, DC: NASW.

Mizrahi, T. & Rosenthal, B. (1993). Managing dynamic tensions in social change coalitions, in Mizrahi, T. & Morrison, J. D. (Eds.), *Community organization and social administration*. New York: The Haworth Press, Inc., pp. 11-40.

Mondros, J. B. & Wilson, Scott M. (1994). *Organizing for power and empowerment*. New York: Columbia University Press.

Montiel, M. & Ortego y Gasca, F. (1992). Chicanos, communities and change, in Rivera, F. G. & Erlich, J. L. (Eds.), *Community organizing in a diverse society.* Boston: Allyn and Bacon. pp. 49-66.

Morales, J. (1992). Community social work with Puerto Rican communities in the United States: One organizer's perspective, in Rivera, F. G. & Erlich, J. L. (Eds.), *Community organizing in a diverse society.* Boston: Allyn and Bacon. pp. 91-112.

Murase, K. (1992). Organizing in the Japanese American community, in Rivera, F. G. & Erlich, J. L. (Eds.), *Community organizing in a diverse society.* Boston: Allyn and Bacon. pp. 159-180.

National Congress for Community Economic Development (1991). *Human investment–Community profits*. Report and recommendations of the Social

Services and Economic Development Task Force. Washington, DC: National Congress for Community Economic Development.

Newstetter, W. I. (1947). The social intergroup work process, in *Proceedings of the National Conference of Social Work.* New York: Columbia University Press, pp. 205-217.

Perlman, R. (1965). Social planning and community organization, in *Encyclopedia of Social Work*, 15th Edition, pp. 1404-1411.

Perlmutter, F. D. (Ed.) (1994). Women & social change: Nonprofits and social policy. Washington, DC: NASW.

Pettit, W. W. (1928). *Case studies in community organization.* New York: Century Co.

Piven, F. F. & Cloward, R. S. (1979). *Poor peoples movements: Why they succeed, how they fail.* New York: Vintage Books.

Plotz, D. A. (1992). *Community problem solving: Case summaries, Volume III.* Washington, DC: Program for Community Problem Solving.

Pray, K. L. M. (1949). *Social work in a revolutionary age.* Philadelphia: University of Pennsylvania Press.

Reisch, M. & Wenocur, S. (1986, March). The future of community organization in social work: Social activism and the politics of profession building. *Social Service Review*, 60 (1) pp. 70-93.

Rivera, F. G. & Erlich, J. L. (Eds.) *Community organizing in a diverse society.* Boston: Allyn and Bacon.

Roberts-DeGennaro, M. (1986). Factors contributing to coalition maintenance. *Journal of Sociology and Social Welfare*, 13, pp. 248-264.

Roberts-DeGennaro, M. (1987). Patterns of exchange relationships in building a coalition. *Administration in Social Work*, 11, pp. 59-67.

Ross, M. G. (1958). *Case histories in community organization.* New York: Harper & Row.

Ross, M. G. (1955). *Community organization: Theory and principles.* New York: Harper & Brothers.

Ross, M. G. with Lappin, B. W. (1967). *Community organization: Theory, principles and practice.* New York: Harper and Row.

Rothman, J. (1964). An analysis of goals and roles in community organization practice. *Social Work* 9(2), pp. 24-31.

Rothman, J. (1995). Approaches to community intervention, Chapter 1 in Rothman, J., Erlich, J. L., & Tropman, J. E. (Eds.), *Strategies of community intervention, Fifth Edition.* Itasca, IL: Peacock, pp. 26-63.

Rothman, J. (March 1994). Expansion of three models of community organization practice, paper presented at the ACOSA Symposium at the CSWE Annual Program Meeting, Atlanta.

Rothman, J. (1974). *Planning & organizing for social change: Action principles from social science research.* New York: Columbia University Press.

Rothman, J. (1979). Three models of community organization practice: Their mixing and phasing, in Cox, F., Erlich, J. L., Rothman, J. and Tropman, J. E. (Eds.) (1987). *Strategies of community organization, Fourth Edition.* Itasca, IL: F.E. Peacock. pp. 25-45.

Rothman, J. (Ed.) (1971). *Promoting social justice in the multigroup society.* New York: Association Press with CSWE.

Rothman, J., Erlich, J. L., & Tropman, J. E. with Cox, F. M. (1995). *Strategies of community intervention, Fifth Edition*. Itasca, IL: Peacock.

Rothman, J. & Zald, M. N. (1985). Planning theory in social work community practice, in Taylor and Roberts (Eds.), *Theory and practice of community social work.* New York: Columbia University Press. pp. 125-153.

Rubin, H. J. & Rubin, I. S. (1992). *Community organizing & development, Second Edition*. New York: Macmillan.

Rubin, H. J. & Rubin, I. S. (1986). *Community organizing & development.* Columbus, OH: Merrill Publishing Co.

Sager, M. (1996). Tyrrell county sustainable development project, presentation to UNC-CH SSW Sustainable Development Class.

Sanderson, E. D. and Polson, R. A. (1939). *Rural community organization*. New York: John Wiley & Sons.

Schwartz, M. (1965). Community organization, in *Encyclopedia of social work*, 15th Edition. Washington, DC: NASW Press.

Shimp, E. C. (1959). The case for a curriculum in community organization for social welfare, in H. L. Lurie (Ed.), *The community organization method in social work education*, Volume IV of the Project Report of the Social Work Curriculum Study. Washington, DC: CSWE, pp. 231-245.

Sieder, V. M. (1947). "The relation of agency and community welfare council structure to community organization," in D. Howard, ed., *Community organization: Its nature and setting*. New York: American Association of Social Workers.

Sieder, V. M. (1950). "The community welfare council and social action" in *Social work in the current scene, 1950. Proceedings of The National Conference of Social Work.* New York: Columbia University Press.

Smith, M. (1979). Concepts of community work: A British view, in Chekki (Ed.), *Community development: Theory and method of planned change*. pp. 47-59.

Steiner, Jesse (1930). *Community organization: A study of its theory and current practice*, Revised edition. New York: Century Co.

Tropman, J. E. (1971). Community welfare councils, in Morris, R. (Editor-in-Chief), *Encyclopedia of social work Sixteenth Edition, Volume I*, pp. 150-156.

Simon, B. L. (1994). *The empowerment tradition in American social work: A history.* New York: Columbia University Press.

Sherrad, T. (1964). *Planned community change in The Social Welfare Forum, 1964: Official Proceedings, 91st Annual Forum National Conference on Social Welfare, Los Angeles, CA, May 24-29.* New York: Columbia University Press.

Solomon, B. B. (1986). *Black empowerment: Social work in oppressed communities*. New York: Columbia.

Staples, L. (1990). Powerful ideas about empowerment. *Administration in Social Work*, 14 (2), pp. 29-42.

Syers, M. (1995). Mary Parker Follett, Biography in Edwards, R. L. (Ed.), *Encyclopedia of social work, Nineteenth Edition*. Washington DC: NASW, p. 2585.

Taylor, S. H. "Community work and social work: The community liaison approach," in Taylor, S. H. & Roberts, R. W. (Eds.). (1985). *Theory and practice of community social work*. New York: Columbia University Press. pp. 179-214.

Taylor, S. H. & Roberts, R. W. (1985). *Theory and practice of community social work*. New York: Columbia University Press.

De Tocqueville, A. (1956). R. D. Heffner (Ed.), *Democracy in america*. New York: Mentor Books.

Tropman, J. E., Erlich, J. L., & Rothman, J. (Eds.) (1995). *Tactics and techniques of community intervention*, Third Edition. Itasca, IL: Peacock.

Van Den Berg, N. & Cooper, L. B. (Eds.). (1986). *Feminist visions for social work*. Washington, DC: NASW.

Vuong, V. and Huynh, J. D. (1992). South East Asians in the United States: A strategy for accelerated and balanced integration, in Rivera, F. G. & Erlich, J. L. (Eds.), *Community organizing in a diverse society*. Boston: Allyn and Bacon. pp. 201-222.

Warren, R. L. (1977). *Social change and human purpose: Toward understanding and action*. Chicago: Rand McNally.

Warren, R. L. (1963). *The community in America*. Chicago: Rand McNally.

Weick, A. & Vandiver, S. T. (Eds.) (1982). *Women, power and change*. Washington, DC: NASW.

Weil, M. & Gamble, D. N. (1995). Community practice models, in Edwards, R. L. (Ed.), *Encyclopedia of social work, Nineteenth Edition*. Washington, DC: NASW, pp. 577-594.

Weil, M. (1995). Women, community and organizing. In Tropman, J. E., Erlich, J. L., & Rothman, J. (Eds.), *Tactics and techniques of community intevention*, Third Edition. Itasca, IL: Peacock. pp. 118-134.

Williams, J. (1987). *Eyes on the prize: America's civil rights years–1954-1965*. New York: Viking Penguin Inc.

Wood, G. G. & Middleman, R. R. (1989). *The structural approach to direct practice in social work*. New York: Columbia University Press.

Wood, J. L. & Jackson, M. (1982). *Social movements: Development, participation, and dynamics*. Belmont, CA: Wadsworth Publishing Co.

Young, W. M. Jr. (1960). Intergroup relations and social work practice in *The Social Welfare Forum, 1960: Official Proceedings, 87th Annual Forum National Conference on Social Welfare Atlantic City NJ, June 5-10*. New York: Columbia University Press.

The Interweaving of Community Intervention Approaches

Jack Rothman, PhD

SUMMARY. This article presents the updated and revised version of the three pronged model of community intervention–locality development, social action, and social planning/policy–introduced in the first edition of *Strategies of Community Intervention* (1968). It provides a recent elaboration of that model into a paradigm of community intervention that illustrates the interweaving of the basic models and the types of interventions that result from the mixed forms. Dilemmas inherent in each core model are analyzed.

KEYWORDS. Community intervention, community practice, community organizing, social action, locality development, social planning and policy.

Jack Rothman is Professor Emeritus of Social Welfare at the University of California, Los Angeles.

Address correspondence to: Jack Rothman, Department of Social Welfare, 247 Dodd Hall, Box 951452, University of California at Los Angeles, Los Angeles, CA 90024-1452.

This paper presents a section of Jack Rothman's "Approaches to Community Intervention" from *Strategies of Community Intervention* (1995), edited by Jack Rothman, John L. Erlich, John E. Tropman, with Fred M. Cox. Reprinted with permission of F.E. Peacock: Itasca, IL.

[Haworth co-indexing entry note]: "The Interweaving of Community Intervention Approaches." Rothman, Jack. Co-published simultaneously in *Journal of Community Practice* (The Haworth Press, Inc.) Vol. 3, No. 3/4, 1996, pp. 69-99; and: *Community Practice: Conceptual Models* (ed: Marie Weil) The Haworth Press, Inc., 1996, pp. 69-99.

Personal Preface by the Author

Not long ago at a conference a colleague asked me why I had never revised the "Three Models" strategy formulation that I had introduced some time back in the late '60s. I managed to give an off hand reply, but thought further about it later. I came to realize that essentially the formulation had suited my purposes as it stood and allowed me to pursue my interests comfortably.

The formulation originally provided a framework for me at a time when there was an enormous amount of confusion and ambiguity about the nature of community intervention. It permitted me to meet my teaching responsibilities and to have a cognitive map for guiding my work generally. The immediate task, it seemed to me, was not to tinker with and refine the niceties of an encompassing theory, but to develop more specific intervention strategies and theoretical constructs dealing with particular issues, processes, and goals. This would require empirical examination of the interactive effects of given variables in the community arena on one another.

My first undertaking was to retrieve and synthesize a large store of existing empirical research knowledge that draws on published studies from diverse social science and professional disciplines (Rothman, 1974). This research utilization exercise using an emergent form of meta-analysis resulted in a series of several hundred empirical generalizations and action hypotheses regarding varied aspects of community intervention.

A next logical step was to select out and field test some of these hypotheses (intervention x will result in outcome y) by having them systematically implemented by practitioners and evaluated by researchers in agency settings. Specific areas of intervention, such as promoting innovation, fostering participation, and changing organizational goals were studied by my colleagues and me in this way (Rothman, Teresa, & Erlich, 1977; Rothman, Erlich, & Teresa, 1976). As practice-oriented researchers, it seemed necessary to present findings in user-friendly handbooks and manuals that field people could readily follow (Rothman, Teresa, & Erlich, 1978). It also seemed appropriate to us to disseminate such information widely to those who might benefit from its availability, drawing on contemporary methods of diffusion and social marketing (Rothman, Teresa, Kay, & Morningstar, 1983).

Through following this interconnected series of steps, a methodology of intervention research (or research and development), was conceived. The methodology was designed to provide a basis for relating research to practice, or more specifically, to offer a comprehensive means to create the tools of intervention and test practice theories (Rothman, 1980; Rothman & Thomas, 1994).

I applied this methodological frame subsequently to other problem areas, in the process developing programmatic techniques for runaway and homeless adolescents (Rothman, 1991) and service modalities for highly vulnerable populations (Rothman, 1992, 1994). The later project involved case management, which constitutes an integrated package of micro and macro practice methods.

Over this time period, conditions in communities had changed in regard to politics, economics, and human service policies. In recent years, questions from students and practitioners about the models schema posed dilemmas that I found it difficult to resolve. My research studies pointed up gaps and uncertainties. The "good enough" conceptual framework was not working as well as it had previously. Community processes had become more complex and variegated, and problems had to be approached differently, more subtly, and with greater penetrability.

What I had seen as community intervention models and ideal types, I began to view increasingly as broader and more loosely defined approaches or modes. Further, they overlap and combine in various admixtures, which can be delineated and identified with specific organizations that provide empirical examples.

This presentation will focus on the mixing and interlinking of strategies, but it would be useful at the outset to very briefly set forth the initial formulation on which it builds. We start with the notion of three basic approaches that include the community-building emphasis of locality development, with its attention to community competency and social integration; the data-based problem-solving orientation of social planning/social policy, with its reliance on expertise; and the advocacy thrust of social action, with its commitment to fundamental change and social justice. Table 1 presents an up-dated visualization of the scheme, showing the relationship between intervention approaches and certain practice variables. The remainder of this discussion is reformulation and expansion of this initial conceptualization.

TABLE 1. Three Community Intervention Approaches According to Selected Practice Variables

	Mode A (Locality Development)	Mode B (Social Planning Policy)	Mode C (Social Action)
1. Goal categories of community action	Community capacity and integration; self-help (process goals)	Problem solving with regard to substantive community problems (task goals)	Shifting of power relationships and resources; basic institutional change (task or process goals)
2. Assumptions concerning community structure and problem conditions	Community eclipsed, anomie; lack of relationships and demographic problem-solving capacities; static traditional community	Substantive social problems, mental and physical health, housing, recreation, etc.	Aggrieved populations, social injustice, deprivation, inequality
3. Basic change strategy	Involving a broad cross section of people in determining and solving their own problems	Gathering data about problems and making decisions on the most logical course of action	Crystallizing issues and mobilizing people to take action against enemy targets
4. Characteristic change tactics and techniques	Consensus: communication among community groups and interests; group discussion	Consensus or conflict	Conflict confrontation, direct action, negotiation
5. Salient practitioner roles	Enabler-catalyst, coordinator; teacher of problem-solving skills and ethical values	Fact gatherer and analyst, program implementer, expediter	Activist advocate: agitator, broker, negotiator, partisan

	Mode A (Locality Development)	Mode B (Social Planning Policy)	Mode C (Social Action)
6. Medium of change	Guiding small, task-oriented groups	Guiding formal organizations and treating data	Guiding mass organizations and political processes
7. Orientation toward power structure(s)	Members of power structure as collaborators in a common venture	Power structure as employers and sponsors	Power structure as external target of action: oppressors to be coerced or overturned
8. Boundary definition of the beneficiary system	Total geographic community	Total community or community segment	Community segment
9. Assumptions regarding interests of community subparts	Common interests or reconcilable differences	Interests reconcilable or in conflict	Conflicting interests which are not easily reconcilable, scarce resources
10. Conception of beneficiaries	Citizens	Consumers	Victims
11. Conception of beneficiary role	Participants in an interactional problem-solving process	Consumers or recipients	Employers, constituents, members
12. Use of Empowerment	Building the capacity of a community to make collaborative and informed decisions; promoting feeling of personal mastery by residents	Finding out from consumers about their needs for service; informing consumers of their service choices	Achieving objective power for beneficiary system-the right and means to impact community decisions; promoting a feeling of mastery by participants

REFERENCES

Rothman, J. (1974). *Planning and organizing for social change: Action guidelines from social science research*. New York: Columbia University Press.

Rothman, J., Erlich, J. L., & Teresa, J. G. (1976). *Promoting innovation and change in organizations and communities: A planning manual*. New York: John Wiley and Sons.

Rothman, J., Teresa, J. G., & Erlich, J. L. (1977). *Developing effective strategies of social intervention: A research and development methodology*. PB-272454 TR-1-RD. Springfield, VA: National Technical Information Service.

Rothman, J., Teresa, J. G., & Erlich, J. L. (1978). *Fostering participation and innovation: Handbook for human service professionals*. Itasca, IL: F.E. Peacock Publishers, Inc. (Formerly *Mastering Systems Intervention Skills*, a publication of the Community Intervention Project, University of Michigan, Ann Arbor, MI.)

Rothman, J. (1980). *Social R & D: Research and development in the human services*. Englewood Cliffs, NJ: Prentice-Hall.

Rothman, J., Teresa, J. G., Kay, T. L., & Morningstar, G. C. (1983). *Marketing human service innovations*. Beverly Hills, CA: Sage Publications.

Rothman, J. (1991). *Runaway and homeless youth: Strengthening services to families and children*. White Plains, NY: Longman.

Rothman, J. (1992). *Guidelines for case management; Putting research to professional use*. Itasca, IL: F.E. Peacock.

Rothman, J., & Thomas, E. J. (Eds.). (1994). *Intervention research: Design and development of human services*. Binghamton, NY: The Haworth Press, Inc.

Rothman, J. (1994). *Practice with highly vulnerable clients: Case management and community-based service*. Englewood Cliffs, NJ: Prentice-Hall.

THE INTERWEAVING OF INTERVENTION APPROACHES

This analysis has attempted to delineate rather distinct and coherent categories of community intervention practice. Alfred North Whitehead offered a rationale for this: "The aim of science is to seek the simplest explanations of complex facts." But while supporting the effort to harness complicated processes, he also alerted us to the underside. We may come to actually believe the original facts are simple because our quest was to arrive at a simplified construction. The French social critic Raymond Aron once spoke of this as *delire logique*–logical delirium. Therefore, Whitehead went on to admonish: "Seek simplicity and distrust it." Following that dictum, we will now reexamine the previous discussion (of intervention modes), bringing to it the eye of the skeptic.

Up until now we have treated each community intervention approach as though it were a rather self-contained ideal-type. That conceptualization is depicted visually in Figure 1.1. Actually, intervention approaches overlap and are used in mixed form in practice. Figure 1.2 reflects broadly the movement toward overlapping.

Practice in any mode may require tactics that are salient in another approach. For example, neighborhood social actionists interested in aiding the homeless may find it necessary to draw up a social plan in order to obtain funding for desired service projects from DHHS (Modes B and C). Or social planners may decide that the most effective way of establishing a viable low-income housing project is to engage potential residents in deciding on the geo-

FIGURE 1.1. Intervention Modes as Ideal-Types

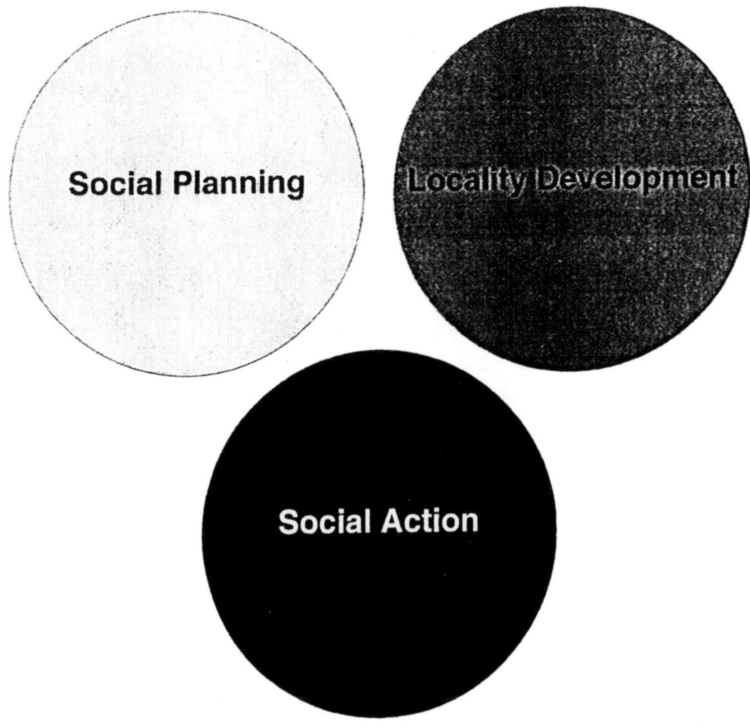

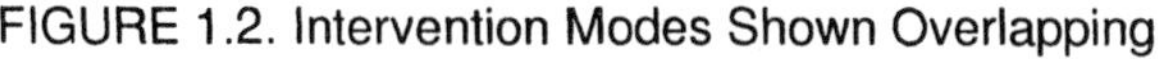
FIGURE 1.2. Intervention Modes Shown Overlapping

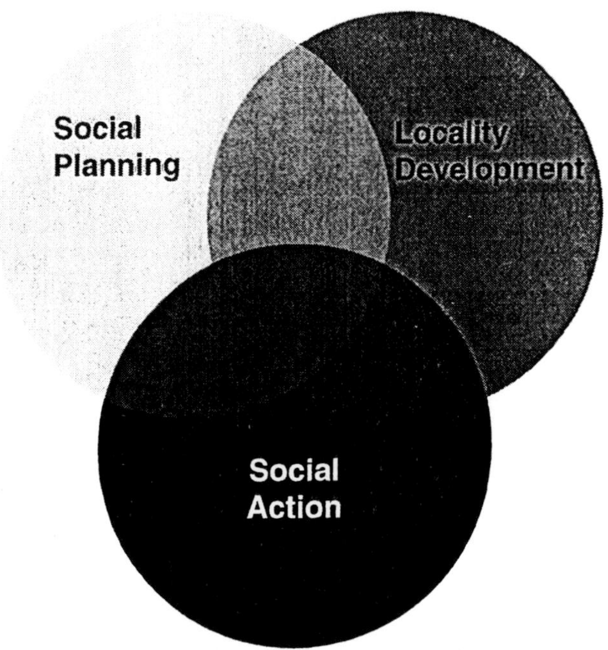

graphic layout and common facilities, and to organize a tenant action council to fight drug pushers (Modes A, B, and C).

A more true-to-life depiction of the character of overlapping is in Figure 1.3. Here we see that the ideal-type modes have a limited scope of frequency and that mixtures of various kinds, along the lines just described, predominate.

To clarify the place of the three practice modes in the overall schema of community intervention, it would be useful to turn to the physical world and the phenomenon of color and its properties. We know that there are three basic colors–red, yellow, and blue. Scrutinizing the properties of these primary colors is valuable because when the properties are mixed they generate an enormous array of hues and shadings. A set of composite secondary colors is yielded when the primary colors are blended in equal proportions. Further

FIGURE 1.3. Overlapping Intervention Modes Showing Estimated Proportional Frequencies of Different Intervention Categories (Modal, Bimodal and Intermixed)

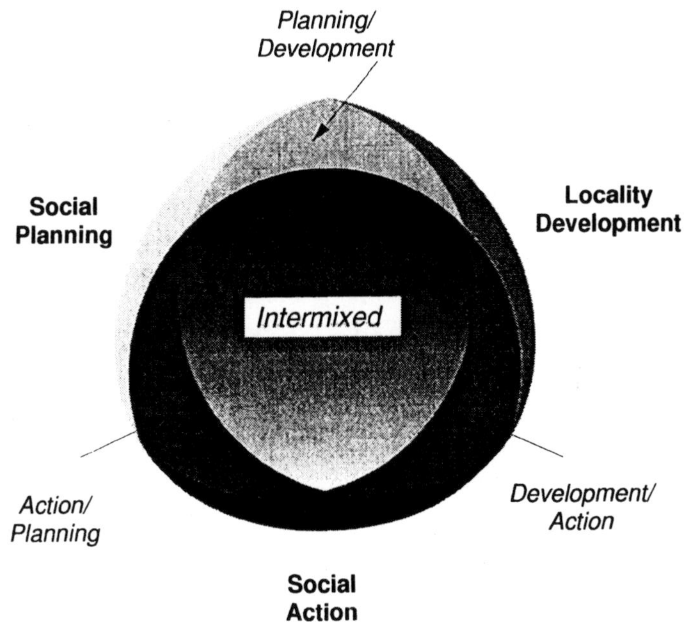

mixtures among all of these result in an almost infinite melange of tones.

Realizing that the analogy is not exact, the three intervention modes can be compared to the three primary colors (but they can only roughly approximate perfect composition in the real world). The basic modes are represented by the outer spheres in Figure 1.3. We can visualize them spawning multiple practice combinations. When two combine, the results are composite bimodal interventions, depicted in the figure by the designations Development/Action, Planning/Development, and Action/Planning. These are analogous to secondary colors.

The center of Figure 1.3 depicts mixed interventions that include a cross-section of variables from all three modes. These combinations involving complex balances of variables are difficult to categorize or even visualize in any succinct fashion.

Just as the primary colors make up only a very small proportion of the total universe of color, the basic intervention modes comprise only a fraction of the world of practice. Predominantly, most practice situations probably entail three-fold mixtures. Bimodal composites, those situations consisting of relatively strong leanings toward two intervention approaches, are probably intermediate in frequency.

These are guesses or loose hypotheses about intricate intervention patterns, rather than verified conclusions. The entire schema is basically a heuristic device that is meant to aid conceptualization. The heuristics, however, have grounded empirical referents and are subject to testing through controlled social research.

COMPOSITE BIMODAL MIXTURES

It would be helpful to further illustrate the overall paradigm in Figure 1.3 and the mixing phenomenon through some examples of the three composite bimodal forms. Note that the composite forms are not uniform in character or coloration, as Figure 1.4 depicts. The mid-area in each composite section of the diagram represents an equally balanced mixing of practice variables from the basic modalities, variables from that mode increasingly predominate in the blend. Myriad mixtures are possible. We will discuss each of the bimodal composites in turn below.

Development/Action in balanced form is portrayed in feminist organizing and in the Freire style of grassroots work. Hyde (1989) indicates that feminist organizing comprises a combination of traits that are traditionally considered feminine with those that are often considered masculine. The feminine aspect includes humanistic qualities such as caring and nurturance, coupled with the use of democratic processes and structures (an emphasis on consensus, the rotating of tasks, and respecting and engaging the skills of all participants). These aspects are all associated with the locality development mode.

At the same time, the feminist organizing perspective is concerned with fundamental cultural and political change–the elimination of patriarchal society. Hyde indicates, "feminist practice is

FIGURE 1.4. Variations Within the Development/Action Mode

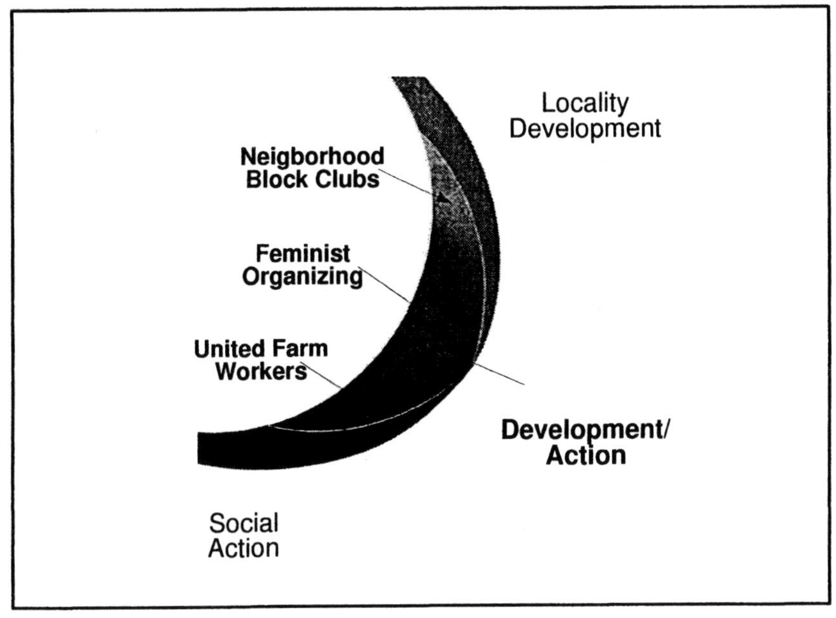

revolutionary. . . . it provides a vision of a radically different society in which the oppressive means of power and privilege are eradicated" (p. 169). These tougher, more militant elements of the practice in the past often have been associated with a masculine posture and the social action intervention mode. Following Hyde's line of analysis, we can say that the feminist organizing perspective, to a considerable degree, is a balanced composite of practice variables involving assumptions and goals of social action joined with the methods of locality development. (See Figure 1.4 for the location of feminist organizing in the Development/Action composite.)

Pablo Freire's work involves a similar blend, in that he has endeavored through an educational approach to empower impoverished peasants in Brazil and Chile to act against the forces of their oppression. He visualizes "education as the practice of freedom," and through "conscientization" seeks, in a sympathetic and enabling manner, to assist illiterate people to see clearly and realistically their objective state of being (Freire, 1974). Fortified with this information, they presumably will gain the motivation and wherewithal to take the steps necessary to transform the closed, unjust societies that repress them. Again, we see the means of locality development wedded to the goals of social action.

The composites we have illustrated represent a somewhat equal mixing of practice variables from Development and Action. They are akin to what is represented by "pure" secondary colors. But the mix might also involve a disproportionate weighting of variables from one or other of the two intervention modes. A composite leaning closer to locality development (see Figure 1.4) is found in Neighborhood Block Clubs. They promote socialization, sharing of information, neighborhood safety watches, mutual aid, and preservation of cherished neighborhood values and landmarks. The overall emphasis is on these Development features. However, when threatened by a porno movie house moving into the area, or the need for a traffic light to protect their children, the organization occasionally swings into a strong and even emotional ad hoc advocacy style.

On the other side of this dual composite stands an organization such as the United Farm Workers, as shown in Figure 1.4. Here the main thrust has been to raise the economic and social well-being of migrant farm workers, using a variety of advocacy measures, such as picketing, marches, and a sustained grape boycott. But there is also a less prominent or visible component that involves mutual aid and community-building among the membership, almost in the form of an extended intraethnic block club. Again, both modes coexist, but in different proportions from the typical block club on the other end of the spectrum.

The Action/Planning composite in balanced form is manifested in the various consumer protection programs of the Ralph Nader organization. This is shown in Figure 1.5, which depicts all the other illustrative organizations mentioned in this presentation. Figure 1.5 will serve as a useful reference guide through the remainder of the discussion. Advocacy in favor of consumer interests is a key thrust with Nader, including tactics that involve media exposure of corporate and governmental abuses, consumer boycotts, legislative campaigns, and the like. At the same time, there is a heavy reliance

FIGURE 1.5. The Paradigm of Community Intervention Showing Examples of Organizational Types for Each Mode of Intervention and Mixed Forms

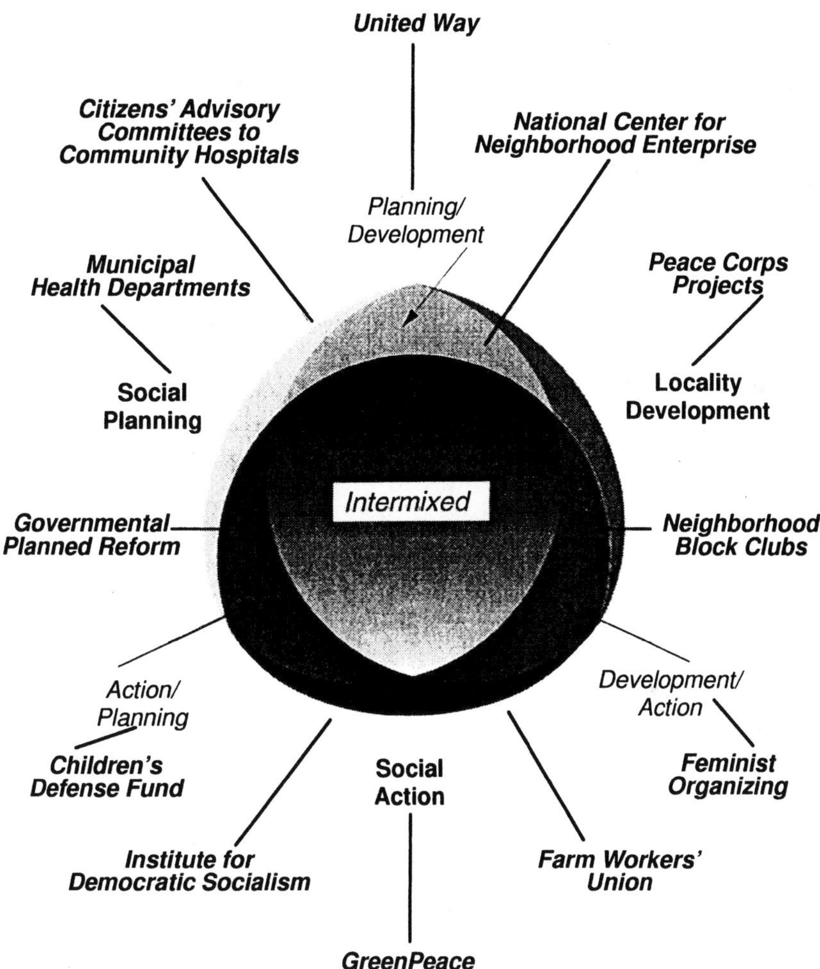

on factual documentation through well-researched and sophisticated reports prepared by expert data analysts and policy specialists. There is also the dissemination of accurate empirical information to consumers so that they can make valid choices. The integration of Action and Planning methods is inseparable. Nader's

Public Citizen organization carries out some grassroots programs–particularly on college campuses–which include a locality development component. But locality development is in pale hue, overall. Another prominent example of a close mix of Action and Planning/Policy is The Children's Defense Fund, a high profile child advocacy organization that uses research data most effectively.

A different type of balanced example is found in municipal-level citizen housing councils. While advocating for more and better housing, consistent with community welfare, these councils have to be prepared to engage in sophisticated interorganizational coordination and negotiation, and to bring to bear the tools and procedures of urban planning professionals, whose analyses and recommendations from within the planning bureaucracy they need to be able to convincingly counter or modify.

Action/Planning with an accent on social action is embodied in organizations on the left that draw up well-formulated policy blueprints for fundamental tax reform, massive low-income housing, and widespread single-payer health services provided under governmental auspices. The groups are essentially geared to social change, but they incorporate data-based reports and policy analyses into their work. The Institute for Democratic Socialism, a "think tank" of the Democratic Socialists of America, is an example. Similar in nature, but pointing to change in another direction (dismantling the welfare state, as an example), are a number of ideologically conservative institutes (the Hoover, for example), commissions, and foundations.

Another example is the area of "advocacy planning" (Davidoff, 1965), whereby grassroots organizations dedicated to change (or blocking intrusive projects) hire a planner or receive pro bono services from a professional, in order to design proposals that can be used with governmental bureaus of planning officials in support of given aims or positions. These planners may serve for only a limited time period or for only one of the many issues being advocated by the organization.

Shifting emphasis toward the planning dimension, Friedman (1987) suggests a role involving a planner/policy analyst firmly ensconced within a governmental structure, where the professional essentially carries out technical planning functions, but with social reform in mind. Friedman notes the role of Rexford Tugwell in Roosevelt's New Deal administration as an example. Robert Moses, in his role during the LaGuardia mayoralty in New York City, would be another. The Koerner Commission functioned similarly, transforming an investigation of urban civil unrest from a focus on social control to issues of equal opportunity. The practitioner's position, methods, and tone are fixed within a governmental bureaucracy, but there is a social advocacy dimension. Friedmann conceives of this government-sponsored planned reform as a distinct fourth intervention mode, in addition to the three we have discussed.

Planning/Development mixtures have a different patterning. The United Way, a convenient balanced example, is dedicated to systematic welfare decision making on the community level with regard to fundraising, budgeting, fund allocation, and coordination of services. However, it places a great deal of stress on citizen participation in these processes. Planning *and* volunteerism are the traditional hallmarks of the organization. Planning for the annual campaign and distributing financial resources to agencies are ongoing activities. But a considerable amount of energy is applied to recruiting community participants (who are most often business and professional elites), training leaders, giving workshops, and holding meetings and conferences of various kinds. Planning and Development are intimately intertwined.

Enterprise/empowerment zones also closely blend these modes of intervention but in a different way. Their aim is to promote community building in inner cities through enhancing the capacity of minority residents to perform in economic and social realms, particularly by starting and running their own businesses. Local initiative and self-reliance are watchwords. But these programs also involve heavy inputs from the outside by corporate and government experts, and the design of elaborate processes to steer a process that is complex and quite technical in nature.

A composite that is weighted toward the planning side is found in citizen advisory committees that are established in the health field by departments of health, community hospitals, and hospital planning councils. These committees have an adjunct role in supporting the basic planning function, which often has a strong technical component. The committees do not ordinarily impact on policy, although they may play some part in policy implementation. They serve to provide legitimization in the community for decisions of planners and administrators; they also have a public relations element. For this reason, energy is applied by the organization to recruiting members, orienting them, and maintaining their bonds. This locality development component is, generally speaking, token rather than substantive in character.

On the other side of the spectrum, an organization such as the National Center for Neighborhood Enterprise is committed to furthering local initiative in urban neighborhoods, as well as seeking to empower poor and minority communities through self-help (while discouraging the means of political insurgency). The Center reflects the work and views of Robert L. Woodson, Sr., who is perhaps the chief organizer of locality development endeavors within African-American communities. In pursuing its goals, the Center actively compiles relevant data and employs the techniques of policy analysts and social planners. These, however, are subsidiary to and in support of the main development thrust.

Taking a different analytical stance now, the character of composite mixes results from the particular configuration of practice variables from each intervention mode. The exact coloration can be influenced by the sheer *number* or volume of variables from either mode of the *types* of variables from each (goals, assumptions, roles, tactics). The *potency* of different types of variables also may have an effect. For example, in feminist organizing, the goal of fundamentally changing gender roles in society is in ascendancy, sometimes dominating the question of tactics (as indicated by existing tactical variations between the position stated by Hyde and that of the radical lesbian movement).

Trimodal mixtures are even more varied than what we have already discussed. An example should suffice to illustrate the general notion. Community welfare planning councils bring social agencies together to share ideas and information, and to strengthen their bonds, in order to become a more successful and integrated service delivery system. The councils also hammer out specific plans and policy frames, in conjunction with the agencies, that are geared to providing more effective and efficient services to community residents. In addition, these organizations actively engage in advocacy, lobbying the city council and the state legislature for more funds and better mandates to meet client needs and expedite agency operations. Chambers of commerce use the same set of intermingled actions on behalf of the business community.

Illustrating intervention mixtures, with all their gradations, can go on endlessly. Examples given here should suffice to demonstrate the basic concept, to generate useful efforts by others, and to fuel critiques of the general information.

DILEMMAS IN EACH INTERVENTION MODE

There are other ways of analyzing the blending of forms of intervention. For each intervention mode we will frame a key issue that confounds the original modal formulation and has implications for expanding and mixing the intervention modes. The dilemmas we will pose spring in part from deliberately positing constructs in ideal or synthetic form, but they arise also from the complex, contentious, constraining, and obdurate social environment in which change agents currently find themselves. In response, practitioners have designed strategies that are more variegated, subtle, flexible, and inventive–and less one-dimensional–than earlier in time.

Locality Development–External Linkages

We have seen that locality development places heavy emphasis on a self-contained local community context. This circumscribed, while holistic, community system is the arena in which features of grassroots initiative, self-help, intimate relationships, and enhanced competency are played out.

A dilemma is that often locality development programs are sponsored and funded by outside entities: municipal (city department of community development); national (The National Service Corps, Campaign for Human Development of the United States Catholic Conference); or international (The World Bank, The World Health Organization). This poses a threat to the conceptual integrity of the formulation. Jacobsen (1990) observes that "much of the initiative for community development actually originates from outside the community, which is a clear violation for the principles of community development" (p. 395).

Vertically linked organizations provide planning and administrative inputs that are hierarchical in nature. They choose the main goals to be pursued, recruit and select staff, train them, set the program emphasis, and establish the rules of practice engagement. These planning elements are vividly portrayed in a description of how the New Zealand central government shifted away from a welfare services policy and designed a local community development approach for the native Maori population (Fleras, 1984).

Local groups are also often linked horizontally at the city or regional level with other similar local groups. Thus, a block club can affiliate with a council of neighborhood block clubs, or a neighborhood citizens association can become part of a citywide council of citizen groups or an interfaith umbrella organization of congregations. Here the coordination and information-sharing aspects of planning play a part, although elements of social action coalition-building may also be involved.

These relationships and entanglements contradict the self-enclosed quality of the original modal formulation. The broader formulation of locality development is shown in Figure 1.6, with the shaded area delineating the original construct.

Social Planning/Policy–Participation

A dilemma in the original social planning concept is that even highly technical planning and policy development that is data-driven and expertise-based often includes elements of participation, in various forms and to varying degrees. The survey by Checkoway (1984) of extant planning endeavors describes a pattern of extensive citizen participation in planning endeavors of municipal departments and of private neighborhood planning organizations. This injects an important element of the locality development approach into the picture.

Political analyst Joel Kropkin observed, in the early Riordan mayoralty in Los Angeles, that there was a danger the new civic leader would lean too heavily on previous corporate experience in his effort to reorganize city government operations and services. In industry, Riordan was able to use soundly conceived technical plans

FIGURE 1.6. Locality Development Intervention Showing Community-Bounded and Externally-Linked Structural Forms (Original Construct is in Shaded Area)

Local and Community-Bounded	Horizontally Linked	Vertically Linked
Neighborhood Councils *Block Clubs* *Self-Help Projects*	*Local Block Groups Affiliated with Regional Councils of Block Clubs* *Coalitions of Local Neighborhood Councils* *Information Clearing Houses*	*Peace Corps Projects* *Church-Sponsored Overseas Development Projects (American Friends Service Committee)* *United Nations Community Development Projects (World Health Organization, World Bank)* *National Service Corps*

"for brokering deals between well-defined and somewhat logical, shareholders and other constituencies." Planning in a community context is different–more fluid and political–says Kropkin, with no evidence that "once a rational plan is developed, support for it will naturally follow." Instead he maintains, it is essential that interests of various kinds be drawn into participation in this process, including municipal unions, churches, grassroots groups, city council members, and others (Kropkin, 1993, pp. 1, 6).

A reformulation of planning that includes the participation dimension is in Figure 1.7. We observe that decision making, as proposed in the original modal formulation, is sometimes concentrated–in the hands of a small group of elite leaders and professional experts (see the shaded area of the figure). Often city departments of child welfare, mental health, housing, and health operate in this way, as do the boards of private agencies like family service organizations, Jewish federations, and boys' clubs.

But planning can entail dispersed decision making, where other than elites alone take part in making judgments and choices. This broader form can involve both *substantive* participation in decision making, and *ancillary*, more peripheral involvement.

First, let us consider substantive activity. Residents and citizens

FIGURE 1.7. Social Planning Intervention Showing Concerted Decision Making and Dispersed Decision Making Involving Various Forms and Degrees of Community Participation (original construct in shaded area)

Concentrated Decision Making	Dispersed Decision Making			
	Substantive Participation in Decisions		Ancillary Participation in Decisions	
City and County Departments of Health, Housing Social Services	United Way Regional Planning Boards	Local Branches of National Service or Planning Organizations–NAACP, Cancer Society	Regional Meetings on Zoning Changes in City Planning	Planners for Neighborhood Halfway Houses
Boards of Voluntary Social Agencies–Family Service, Citizens' Planning, and Housing Councils	Free Clinics		Locally Conducted Congressional Hearings	Real Estate Developers of Shopping Malls and Housing Complexes, Environmental Impact Reports
	OEO projects–"Maximum Feasible Participation"	Federal Program Implementation in the States–Title XX		

can join in policy decisions of a basic nature, or they take part in *implementation decisions* that relate to carrying out programs that grow out of policy decisions by others. The OEO "War on Poverty" spawned a multitude of grassroots organizations where "maximum feasible participation" at the highest policy-making levels was emphasized. Free clinics providing health services to low-income ill people have traditionally encouraged such participation. The United Way's Regional Planning Councils attempt to involve local residents in allocation and program decisions affecting the area.

Substantive implementation decisions, within established policy parameters, are frequently given over to members of local branches of national organizations, such as the American Cancer Society, The Urban League, League of Women Voters, and so forth. Federal legislation, such as Title XX, has often left discretion for implementation in the hands of the states, counties, or municipalities.

Second, ancillary participation can be *facilitative* or *symbolic.* The facilitative form draws residents into the decision-making process by seeking their reactions to proposals, or asking for their advice. It may also entail providing information about impending changes in order to prepare people for them, thereby reducing stress or disruption in their lives. Regional meetings called by city planning departments to announce zoning changes or to ask people for their opinions about these changes are an example. Local hearings conducted by Congress or a city council are another, as are hearings related to environmental impact studies.

Symbolic participation serves to provide the appearance or aura of participation, but not its actuality. The aim is cooperation, whereby the opposition is won over or "cooled out." Real estate developers and housing officials often use this approach in trying to influence residents to accept a new project, as do social planners who attempt to establish group living "halfway houses" in urban neighborhoods for the mentally ill, delinquent adolescents, the homeless, and other vulnerable groups.

There is a tendency among human service professionals to instinctively reject the use of symbolic forms of participation, particularly when these are applied to them and their clients. There are, of course, vital ethical objections to the deceptive quality of this tactic but the question is intellectually complex.

Brager, Specht and Torczyner (1987) address this issue in a penetrating discussion, taking the view that "manipulation is an unavoidable component of professional behavior" and that "political maneuvering" is inevitable in community intervention (p. 321). In seeking to advance interests and well-being of those we seek to benefit, when facing inhospitable or potentially damaging actions by others, the practitioner is obligated to "employ artfulness in inducing desired attitudinal or behavioral outcome in others" (p. 317). The foes of our allies and constituents use powerful tools of accepted political in-fighting that challenge our capability to provide protection and nurturance. Brager and his associates recognize the importance and delicacy of this issue, and they delineate a set of factors to be weighed carefully in arriving at ethically sound conclusions about tactics. At the same time, they resist discarding the "planned ambiguity" tactic of symbolic participation, which, if it occurred, might mean abandoning to the winds of political fortune in pluralistic American communities the possibility of establishing group homes for the homeless and the mentally ill.

Social Action–Multiple Actors and Conventional Tactics

Social action is more complicated than the original model conveyed, as reflected in studies that found it to have complex qualities. For example, Cnaan and Rothman (1986) in a factor analysis inquiry discovered that planning and development can be explained through a single, consistent factor. However, social action comprised two or more factors, which were difficult to identify with clarity.

There are three dimensions that probably account for this complexity (see Figure 1.8). The original formulation did not take into account, and did not differentiate, the two essentially different types of goals of this intervention mode. These include radical change goals that aim at fundamental alterations in society or specific policies or institutions within it, and more normative or reformist change goals that aim at incremental alterations. This is a basic context within which social action needs to be understood.

It is difficult to delineate precisely the division between radical and normative goal changes in social action. Radical change suggests breadth of alteration in the society and culture. Examples of this thrust include organizations that militate to eradicate racism or to transform the relationship between the races (as with the Nation of Islam), or to change the basic economic system of the country (as with the Democratic Socialists of America). However, a change that on the surface seems modest can have a broad impact. As an example, changing regulations about what can appear on TV, or the tone of presentation, can have a rippling effect throughout the entire culture because of the widespread influence of the media.

In addition, fundamental change can be narrow and deep rather than wide in scope. The aim may be to alter a specific law or specific sphere of living in a radical way. As an example, the Pro-Life movement focuses on the single issue of abortion legislation, but is interested in drastically overturning existing legal arrangements rather than adjusting or tampering with them. Because of the saliency of the issue, the change being advocated would be seen by many as fundamental, and a deep threat.

FIGURE 1.8. Social Action Intervention Divided by Type of Goal and Further Differentiated by Tactical Means and the Composition of the Action Constituency (Original Construct in the Shaded Area)

MEANS		GOALS: **Radical** Fundamental	GOALS: **Normative** Incremental
Radical Disruptive Tactics	Disadvantaged Parties Mainly	American Indian Movement (AIM) ACT-UP	Industrial Areas Foundation Tenant Action Organizations
	Multiple Parties	Greenpeace The 60s Student and Anti-War Movements (SDS)	Ad Hoc Protests by Alliance for the Mentally Ill Animal Rights Groups
Normative Conventional Tactics	Disadvantaged Parties Mainly	Nation of Islam Center for Third World Organizing	La Raza American Association of Retired Persons
	Multiple Parties	Democratic Socialists of America Wms' Intnl League for Pce and Fdm	Childens' Defense Fund Coalition for the Homeless

Alternatively, radical change can be accomplished through a particular combination of breadth and depth that in aggregate goes beyond incrementalism. The precise calculus of this combination is elusive, but the possibility of it occurring seems plausible.

In any case, it is difficult to establish a firm dividing line between fundamental and incremental change, partly because incremental change is sometimes carried out as a strategic step leading to fundamental change. The extremes of each are easy enough to discern (the Communist Party as compared to the League of Women Voters); it is pinpointing the middle border that separates the tendencies that is vexing.

Two other dimensions beside goal categories suggest revisions rather than additions to the original formulation. One of these concerns the constituency action system for the change effort. Going back to the sixties, social action movements focused on the disadvantaged or aggrieved group only as the vehicle of social change, as with the Black Panthers, AIM (American Indian Movement), La Raza, gay and lesbian groups and others, playing out the politics of identity. Going it alone was a way of ensuring that the fundamental interests of the group were safeguarded, that outsiders who might take over were contained, and group self-empowerment was promoted. This was the outlook incorporated within the original modal formulation.

Contemporary "new movement" organizing is seeking to become broader, more ecumenical. Fisher and Kling (1991) speak in support of "a more consciously ideological politics. New formations and groupings will only make community mobilization stronger. . . . an explicitly challenging ideology is necessary if community movements are not to remain bound by the limits of personalized and localized consciousness" (p. 81). Advocacy groups across class and ethnic lines are forming, focused on environmental protection, crime prevention, neighborhood preservation, animal rights, and health issues. These new groupings and alliances involve community-building methods for achieving cohesion and continuity. Not only are the economically oppressed organizing to act on their own behalf, but, in addition, middle-class aggrieved persons, including right-wing activists and the Ross Perot movement, are involved in victim rights, tax reduction, Pro-Life, government reorganization, and school reform efforts. The expanded constituencies include linkages and coalitions by grassroots groups that are national in scope (Flacks, 1990).

The additional dimension is tactical in nature. Action groups have been characterized by their reliance on aggressive and abrasive advocacy measures, which was reflected in the original formulation. More recently, tactics have been refined and diversified.

They are more normative in quality, utilizing conventional political maneuvers.

Many community organizers today cite a trend toward pragmatism that emphasizes electoral politics, consensus building, data collection and research, and the use of political and administrative channels. Confrontational tactics, while sometimes required, are considered ineffective in many cases. Although sit-in and demonstrations have succeeded in creating awareness of problems, administrators and officials also have learned how to defuse them (Hiratsuka, 1990, p. 3).

These new social action elements suggest the inclusion of practice variables from the other intervention modes. For example, conventional advocacy methods, such as factual documentation of environmental despoilment, include data-based techniques from planning and policy practice. Community-building within and among different advocacy constituencies brings to bear locality development practice.

These elements of social action are tied together and systematized in Figure 1.8. The top two shaded cells encompass the original intervention mode, and the additional six are expanded representations of the advocacy strategy. Each cell incorporates a different form of the admixture of: type of goal (radical/normative), and type of constituency action system (disadvantaged parties mainly/multiple parties). Examples are provided for each of these social action amalgams. The information is essentially self-evident and does not require extended explication.

PHASING, VALUES, AND PRACTICE OPTIONS

The broad approaches, and sets of practice variables within them, offer a range of interrelated possibilities for designing intervention strategies. The point has been stated by Gurin (1966) as follows:

> Our field studies have produced voluminous evidence that (various) roles are needed, but not always at the same time and place. The challenging problem, on which we have made a bare beginning, is to define more clearly the specific conditions under which one or another or still other types of practice

> are appropriate. The skill we shall need in the practitioner of the future is the skill of making a situational diagnosis and analysis that will lead him to a proper choice of the methods most appropriate to the task at hand. (p. 30)

In addition to mixing approaches as discussed, there is a phasing relationship among them. A given change project may begin in one mode and then, at a later stage, move into another. For example, as a social action organization achieves success and attains resources, it may find that it can function most efficiently out of a social planning mode. The labor union movement, to a degree, demonstrates this type of phasing. As organizational growth and viability are achieved, headquarters operations (for example, the teamsters or UAW) become larger, more bureaucratized, and more technical, and social policy and administrative factors become more salient. The practitioner needs to be attuned to appropriate transition points in applying alternative modes.

As practitioners phase through their own careers, there will be demands to emphasize one or another modality. Historically, circumstances and preferences change, resulting in shifts in professional fashion and the employment requisites of agencies. For this reason, it is useful for practitioners to be broadly prepared, with the full range of competencies tucked into their professional portfolio.

Locality development was in vogue in the quiescent 1950s, when interactive, enabling practice was considered the quintessence of professionalism (Pray, 1947; Newstetter, 1947). Planning/policy was important during the Charity Organization Society and Community Chest and Council movements of the 1920s, as an aspect of emergent social work institution building. This mode came to the fore again during the New Deal spurt of policy development and program organization intended to cope with the Great Depression. It was called upon again in the Nixon and Reagan-Bush times of policy reversal and program curtailment, where efforts to promote efficiency, scrupulous evaluation, and cost containment were given prominence. Social action had its heyday during the roiling 1960s, and also in the early years of the century when progressives were advocating for legislation on child labor, workmans' compensation, and housing and municipal reform. Cycles in the relative rise and fall of different intervention modes will doubtless continue in the periods ahead.

In the past, professional actions and conceptualizations were often constrained by particular value orientations to practice–for example, acceptance of only collaborative, nondirective practice (Pray, 1947). Alinsky followers derided all others as "sell-outs," while planners were often disdainful of militants for fomenting disorder and antagonism. The current outlook, however, is more accepting of varying value orientations. An examination of empirical findings on professional values leads to the conclusion that "human service professions do not appear to be highly integrated with regard to the existence of a delimited, uniformly accepted value system" (Rothman, 1974, p. 100). The approaches suggested in this presentation are in the spirit of such a position.

The locality development practitioner will likely cherish values that emphasize harmony and communication in human affairs; the planner/policy specialist will give priority to rationality; the social actionist will build on commitments embracing social justice. Each of these value orientations finds justification in the traditions of the human service professions. It would be difficult to claim monopoly status for any one or other. Indeed, contemporary thinking suggests that values are plural and conflicting, and may well come in pairs of divergent commitments (Tropman, 1984). Mixing occurs on those frequent occasions when more than one value is being pursued at a given time.

The various intervention approaches can all be applied in a way to pursue values conducive to positive social change and human betterment. Our position accepts the validity of each of the stated value postures and encourages their interrelated employment.

Values aside, the intervention modes have to draw from one another because of the inherent functional limitations within each. Planning and policy initiatives have created worthy programs, particularly when pushed by the other two modes, but have accomplished little in redistributing wealth and power or in preventing the victimization of the have-nots. They have typically concealed the vested interests of the professionals and failed to address the widespread alienation of society. Locality development has had its successes in countering isolation and depersonalization in specific places, but not in removing the social conditions that continue to generate anomie and inequality. Social action has confronted power and economic inequities in some measure at the local level, but has not had sufficient potency to cope with larger national power issues or to shape a strategy to rehumanize those it cannot defeat. Each modality alone faces obstacles that the others can contribute to addressing.

Another reason for seeking new configurations of action is that, at the highest societal levels, established institutions and modes of operating are showing grave defects. Eastern European communism, with its outrageous tyrannies and rigidities, has collapsed from within and left a widespread landscape of upheaval and turmoil. But the Western market-dominated countries who are now the only game in town, are saddled with the cruel by-products of an acquisitive ethic, and they display persistent pathologies of economic and social disparity, industrial decay, recurring joblessness, cultural decline, racism, and anomie–to use the short list.

New social forms are called for that combine the liberal ideal of political democracy and the socialist ideal of economic democracy, ensuring a balance of liberty and equality in both spheres. Barbara Ehrenreich (1993) has stated the challenge aptly:

> We must outline how we believe that the community of human beings can live together more equitably and peacefully than it does now. *The vision has to be a vision beyond capitalism, with its inevitable economic injustice. This is a time when people looking for change don't have some kind of precise model to inform that struggle for change.* Everyone has some responsibility to start imagining, dreaming, inventing and visualizing the kind of future we would like.

This discussion prompts us to look back at Table 1.1, the listing of practice variables across intervention modes, and read it in a different light now. The table, in aggregate, provides a repertoire of practice options, for flexible application. Each of the thirty-six cells describes an analytical or behavioral intervention initiative. (This is not a complete enumeration of the possibilities by any means, but it is a suggestive one.) The practice options, when used critically and selectively, can provide vital components to interweave creatively into the design of strategy.

This moves us toward a contingency formulation where practitioners of any stripe have a greater range in selecting, then mixing and phasing, components of intervention. An important next step is to identify a set of situational criteria to inform such tactical packaging. A number of social parameters of the situation readily come to mind, among them the type of change goal and its scope, the quality of constituency leadership, availability of knowledge regarding relevant problems and solutions, the extent and character of resistance, the degree of financial and other resource support at hand, and stage of development of the action system.

There is a need for research concerning which situational criteria, or clusters among them, are most critical for strategy development. Beyond that, it would be useful to study how these criteria specifically inform the selection and meshing of practice options from the repertoire of intervention components, in the interests of designing change strategies with greater impact.

In summary, the goal of this piece has been to lay open and chart a multifaceted change process that plays a large role in inducing the progressive development of society. Historically, what humans have been able to capture cognitively, they often have been able to master behaviorally–which is a reason for persisting in the endeavor. However, there are no panaceas inherent in this text. The world is an unpredictable place, and humans have struggled through time to gain greater control over and better their social environs. One can only believe and hope that a sound, informed analysis coupled with disciplined action will provide some increment of probability beyond intuitive strivings. Through systematic evaluation and other research we can hone our techniques and monitor our results, thereby learning cumulatively from experience and improving our record.

Such efforts are analogous to the realm of interpersonal helping in psychotherapy. It is assumed that use of theory and tested practice will improve on the natural advice and support that neighbors and family provide to one another. Still despite the best efforts of dedicated therapists some clients remain mired in despair and confusion. Those of us in the human services hold the limited aspiration that, to some unknown degree, what we do will enhance the probability that beneficial results will come to pass.

The sharpening of change methods is an endless and evolving process. The mental skirmishing involved in this revision of an earlier construct is captured in T. S. Eliot's (1943) wise and edifying words:

> We shall not cease from exploration.
> And the end of all our exploring will
> be to arrive where we started and know
> the place for the first time.

From that ground, naturally, the exploration begins anew.

REFERENCES

Brager, G., Specht, H., & Torczyner, J. L. (1987). *Community organizing* (2d ed.). New York: Columbia University Press.

Checkoway, B. (1984). Two Types of Planning in Neighborhoods. *Journal of Planning Education and Research*, *2*, 102-109.

Cnaan, R. A., & Rothman, J. (1986). Conceptualizing community intervention: An empirical test of "three models" of community organization. *Administration in Social Work*, *10*(3), 41-55.

Davidoff, P. (1965). Advocacy and pluralism in planning. *Journal of the American Institute of Planners*, *31*(4), 331-37.

Ehrenreich, B. (1993). From a letter to the membership of Democratic Socialists of America, dated December 1, 1993, New York.

Eliot, T. S. (1943). Little Gidding in *The Four Quartets*. New York: Harcourt, Braca.

Fisher, R., & Kling, J. (1991). Popular mobilization in the 1990s: Prospects for the new social movements. *New Politics*, *3*, 71-84

Flacks, D. (Fall 1990). The Revolution of Citizenship. *Social Policy.* New York: Social Policy Corporation, 37-50.

Fleras, A. J. (1984). From Social Welfare to Community Development: Maori Policy and the Department of Maori Affairs in New Zealand. *Community Development Journal*, *19*, 32-39.

Freire, P. (1974). *Education: The practice of freedom*. London: Writers and Readers Publishing Cooperative.

Friedman, J. (1987). *Planning in the public domain: From knowledge to action.* Princeton, NJ: Princeton University Press.

Gurin, A. (1966). *Current issues in community organization practice and education*. Brandeis University Reprint Series, No. 21, p. 30. Florence Heller Graduate School for Advanced Studies in Social Welfare.

Hiratsuka, J. (1990, September). *Community organization: Assembling power.* NASW News.

Hyde, C. (1989). A feminist model for macro-practice: Promises and problems. In Y. Hasenfeld (Ed.), *Administrative leadership in the social services: The next challenge* (pp. 145-181). New York: The Haworth Press, Inc.

Jacobsen, M. (1990). Working with communities. In H. W. Johnson (Ed.), *The social services: An introduction* (3rd ed.) (pp. 385-403). Itasca, IL: F.E. Peacock.

Kropkin, J. (1993, December 19). Riordan's next challenge: Become the political man. *Los Angeles Times*, pp. M1, M6.

Newstetter, W. I. (1947). The social intergroup work process. *Proceedings, National Conference of Social Work*, pp. 205-17. New York: Columbia University Press.

Pray, K. L. M. (1947). When is community organization social work practice? *Proceedings, National Conference of Social Work.* New York: Columbia University Press.

Rothman, J. (1974). *Planning and organizing for social change: Action principles from social science research.* New York: Columbia University Press.

Tropman, J. E. (1984). Value conflict in decision-making. In F. M. Cox et al., *Tactics and techniques of community practice, 2nd ed.* Itasca, IL: F.E. Peacock.

Modelling Community Work: An Analytic Framework for Practice

Ann Jeffries, CSW, MPA

SUMMARY. This paper argues that the most useful aspect of Rothman's development of his models for community practice back in 1968 was his specification of the variables which he used to differentiate between "three important orientations to deliberate or purposive community change in contemporary American communities, both urban and rural, and overseas" (Rothman, 1970, p. 21). While Rothman referred to these three orientations as Models A, B, and C, my contention has been that they would be described more accurately as approaches to practice which are adopted as the outcome of modelling activity using the variables Rothman identified. Indeed it is to the point that Rothman now refers to these as "modes." Yet, ironically, this core feature of Rothman's work on modelling community practice is largely overlooked in subsequent literature on models even though it is this aspect which is an invaluable tool for practice, especially for students embarking on placement or on their first job.

This paper starts from the premise that a model is a simplification of reality that is intended to order and clarify our perception of that reality while still encapsulating its essential characteristics. To have analytical value a model should specify key variables to be considered in assessing a situation in order to develop and evaluate possible

Ann Jeffries is Principle Lecturer and Head of the Department of Social Policy and Social Work at the University of Plymouth in the United Kingdom.

Address correspondence to: Ann Jeffries, Department of Social Policy and Social Work, University of Plymouth, Drake Circus, Plymouth, Devon PL4 8AA, United Kingdom.

[Haworth co-indexing entry note]: "Modelling Community Work: An Analytic Framework for Practice." Jeffries, Ann. Co-published simultaneously in *Journal of Community Practice* (The Haworth Press, Inc.) Vol. 3, No. 3/4, 1996, pp. 101-125; and: *Community Practice: Conceptual Models* (ed: Marie Weil) The Haworth Press, Inc., 1996, pp. 101-125. Single or multiple copies of this article are available for a fee from The Haworth Document Delivery Service [1-800-342-9678, 9:00 a.m. - 5:00 p.m. (EST). E-mail address: getinfo@haworth.com].

action plans. Thus a model should enable prediction of likely outcomes if a particular plan of action is pursued. The paper starts, therefore, by refining the variables identified by Rothman in order to frame them as a model that can hold Rothman's Three Core Modes of Community Intervention. It is proposed that, with some refinement to take account of the insights from further theoretical and practice developments, this can also serve as a simple diagnostic tool to enable analysis by contemporary community workers.

The outcome such analysis seeks is the specification of a basic orientation to practice and thus to the clarification of the strategies, roles and skills that are likely to be most useful given the particular approach chosen. The paper indicates how different theoretical perspectives, as well as approaches and strategies that have been identified since Rothman's original work, inform or fit into the proposed four-square model. In short the paper illustrates how an approach analogous to that employed by Rothman is still essential for reflexive community work. *[Article copies available for a fee from The Haworth Document Delivery Service: 1-800-342-9678. E-mail address: getinfo@haworth.com]*

CORE FEATURES OF ROTHMAN'S MODELS

Rothman's identification of three models of community organisation practice has permeated the community work literature on both sides of the Atlantic. Whatever the subsequent critique, locality development (which in the U.K. is commonly referred to as community development in recognition that 'community' is a more multi-dimensional concept than 'locality' implies), social action and social planning are the common starting points. Yet ironically the purpose, and for me the core feature of Rothman's analysis, is largely overlooked in the literature.

At the end of his chapter in the original 1970 edition of *Strategies of Community Organisation*, Jack Rothman focused on the implications of his discussion of the three models for community practice. Firstly, he stated *"it is important for a practitioner immersed in the organizational and methodological vortex of one of these models to be aware of 'his' grounding. . . . In this way 'he' may perform appropriately, consistent with the expectations of other relevant actors."* Secondly, and of crucial importance in my mind, Rothman wrote: *"the practitioner may be in a position to create a model of action to deal with specific problems."* He then illustrated briefly some "rule-of-thumb guidelines" for assessing situations in light of the variables he had painstakingly outlined in the bulk of the chapter. Rothman concluded:

> *By assessing when one or another mode of action is or is not appropriate, the practitioner takes an analytical, problem-solving stand and does not become the captive of a particular ideological or methodological approach to practice. (p. 35)*

Incidentally for me the latter phrase of that quotation means that this sort of analysis is essential whatever one's ideological orientation, not that an ideological orientation is necessarily problematic. The Association of Community Workers in Britain warns against imposing one's own or one's employing agency's ideological convictions on to communities; however, it also makes clear that it is essential to have a commitment to social justice with which to underpin praxis. Likewise, Weil and Gamble (1995) note that one of the objectives of community practice is "to infuse the social planning process with a concern for social justice" (p. 580).

While Rothman sees a practice that is now "more accepting of varying value orientations" (Rothman, this volume, p. 95), such a statement rings alarm bells for social and community workers in the U.K., who have a professional commitment to a clear anti-oppressive value base. As Weil and Gamble (1995) imply, the community worker opting for the 'rational planner' mode can be just as committed to social justice as the social activist. It is their analysis of the best way to proceed that should vary in accordance with the varying circumstances. Certainly the range of strategies and roles relevant to achieving change and empowering people in the process has expanded. Likewise, the extent of change sought and the degree of empowerment in a given situation will vary, but the values underpinning professional practice do not change.

While community work in the U.S.A. is contained within a broader concept of social work and is built on pluralist assumptions, it is my contention that a downside to the once vigorous socialist strand in British community work is that it partly blinded us to the pertinence of other perspectives. In this sense Rothman is right, in that on both sides of the Atlantic perhaps "professional actions and conceptionalizations were often constrained" (this volume, p. 45), but, I would suggest, by political ideology more than by core values. Perhaps it was this that has resulted in the analytical edge that Rothman brought to his work on models being largely overlooked, along with the impetus to build on his work in light of insights gained from feminist analysis and from the organising experience from various new social movements. It is my contention that this sort of analysis, informed by the rich variety of theoretical perspectives that are available to us now but underpinned with a clear anti-oppressive value base, is the key to effective practice.

SUBSEQUENT DEVELOPMENTS

Much of the subsequent literature in regard to models sidesteps the issue of their use as an analytic process, concentrating on describing variations of the approaches delineated by Rothman (this volume, pp. 69-99; Thomas, 1983; Popple, this volume, pp. 147-180), or by focusing on specific strategies for achieving change (e.g., Checkoway, 1995). Of course the former is useful both in aiding understanding of the development and diverse applications of community work in response to particular funding opportunities or organisational realities, and also in highlighting strategies and community worker roles associated with each approach. Likewise, Checkoway (1995), who does suggest that one keep a simple question to the forefront when deciding on a strategy, namely: "will it empower the community?" draws on wide experience to identify six core strategies, but does he adequately address *how* community workers actually go about assessing whether a particular strategy is the optimum for their situation?

Weil and Gamble provide a more comprehensive analysis in their description of "a new constellation of eight basic models of community practice" (1995, p. 580). Like Rothman their models are based on research on current practice as well as on literature surveys. They differentiate between these models on the basis of five comparative characteristics whereas Rothman lists twelve practice variables. They note that these eight basic models "illustrate the kinds of organizations that exist in the 1990s." Naturally their focus is on the U.S.A., just as Popple's focus is on the U.K. Having lived and worked on both sides of the Atlantic I have been interested in developing a model that has 'goodness of fit' for community practice in general, for then I suggest we will be closer to identifying the crux of what the work is about.

Whatever Rothman's intentions, his work has been used chiefly to differentiate, like Weil and Gamble do, between different approaches to community practice. The focus is on the practice. In this paper my intention is to start at the other end, so to speak. My concern has been to enable students and community activists to begin to make sense of particular community dynamics in order to develop more effective ways to engage with whatever are the pressing issues of concern and to do so in a way that promotes the chances of both long-term and fundamental improvement in the community's quality of and approach to communal life, building a more just and empowering society and thus contributing to the feminist vision of a transformed society.

Indeed as Weil and Gamble note: *"The current realities of practice reveal a complex and interconnected set of models for community practice" (p. 580).* It is this which Rothman recognises in his latest, more elaborate and inclusive paradigm. The danger is that in trying to do justice to the multi-dimensionality of community organising, or in trying to illustrate the various ways in which core approaches may combine and overlap, we lose the simplicity which is the beauty and the potential of modelling. My intention in this paper, therefore, is to present a refined and simplified model for analysing the community situation *as a means for community workers to choose* both an overall approach to practice in particular circumstances and also as tool to develop, phase and assess alternative strategies. It is my contention that the relevance of various modes of community practice can be aided by use of this modelling frame.

PURPOSE OF A MODEL

To have analytic value a model must enable us to abstract the essential elements from complex situations. The intention is to order and clarify our understanding of the situation and facilitate the prediction of likely outcomes if particular actions are undertaken. Inevitably this results in simplification of highly complex situations. A good model will give scope also for recognition of this complexity by reflecting typical ways in which core approaches may overlap or may need to be combined and under what circumstances. This is the challenge Rothman subsequently set himself in the work summarised in this volume. My concern is that it also retain utility in the day to day bustle of community work. Nevertheless the starting point is to identify key variables to be considered in assessing a situation in order to assess how best to approach the work.

IDENTIFICATION OF CORE VARIABLES

It is interesting that in his revised typology of community intervention, Rothman only makes minor modifications to the core variables he used as the basis for differentiating between practice modes. This fits with my experience of applying Rothman's model to community work in the U.S.A., Canada, and the U.K. Using these variables as a frame can enable practitioners to more quickly make sense of the multi-dimensionality of community situations and of the welter of practice possibilities that come under the general community organizing (U.S.A.) or community work (U.K.) umbrella.

Rothman summarised his twelve core variables in Table 1, the latest version of which is found in this volume. For use as an analytic tool by busy practitioners this is a long and rather unwieldy list. To have value for practice I have found it helpful to group these variables. In the first group are those that can be used for a broad analysis of the community situation and thus for an assessment, in general terms, of the likely scope for the work. This includes the determination of realistic overall goals and thus the basic orientation or approach to take to work in the particular community. A further set of variables relate to the identification for each approach of realistic objectives, an effective range of strategies and suitable roles for both community members and the worker in these circumstances. Rothman's presentation of the relationship of the variables to his three practice modes are *the outcome* of this modelling process, so in the main the first page of his table covers what I would consider to be the second order of variables, namely the variables that relate to strategies, tactics, roles and methods. (See variables 3,4,5,6, Table 1.)

However, to identify the optimum practice mode at any given time it is first necessary to ascertain how a given community fares in terms of four more fundamental variables:

a. the community's relationship to the *power structures* that impact upon them;
   –Rothman's variables 7 and 10.
b. *community circumstances* (including dominant attitudes about the community; level of socio-political awareness in the community and extent of organisation);
   –Rothman's variables 2, 9 and 11.
c. *needs, problems and strengths* in the community (including available resources)
   –Rothman's variables 1 and 12.
d. the basis on which workers are involved: *agency and/or worker mandate.*
   –Rothman's variables 11 and 12.

Answers to these questions will enable those involved to size up the extent of change that is needed; its feasibility given the resources likely to be available to the community; the likely resistance to or support for such change both from within the community and from powerful decision makers who could be involved; and how much scope the community and the workers have to make decisions about actions needed to achieve that change, either through participation in organised decision-making processes or through community organisations–in other words the community's state of empowerment. A simple four-square diagramme[1] can assist and illustrate this analysis.

THE FOUR-SQUARE MODEL OF COMMUNITY PRACTICE

On one dimension the community situation can be assessed in terms of the extent of change needed in attitudes, structures, policies and/or the distribution of resources. This can be envisioned as a continuum in which the work called for ranges from improving the status quo, such as better access to, or coordination of, services that address felt needs (which one would expect to be supported, if under-resourced, by local authorities, agencies and organisations) to a radical challenge to authorities, arising from experiences of disenfranchisement or perceived structural injustices, that will require major change. This dimension is illustrated below as the vertical *change axis.*

On the horizontal dimension one can assess the attitudes to and readiness for the community to be involved in decision-making and ownership of any action undertaken. This is envisioned as a continuum stretching between elite decision making at one end through consultation and efforts to promote participation to community decision making at the other–or from powerlessness to empowerment. Thus it is referred to as the *empowerment axis.*

These two dimensions reflect the dual focus in community work on "purposeful community change" (Rothman, 1995, p. 45) on the one hand, and on the other hand on how that change is brought about, namely "by people at the community level" (Rothman, 1995, p. 45). However, that is not the whole story and by modelling this as a continuum the variation in both those dimensions is kept to the forefront of analysis. As Rothman himself stresses in his latest work on Social Planning/Policy–Participation, "We observe that decision making, as proposed in the original modal formulation, is sometimes concentrated–in the hands of a small group of elite leaders and professional experts rather than in the hands of community members." Then in between these two extremes on the decision-making continuum can be found a range of varying degrees of collaborative/participative decision-making. Intersect the two dimensions and the following model is suggested (see Figure 1).

Work that falls into the top two quadrants (A and B) could be expected commonly to be regarded as reasonably legitimate, hence it would not be expected to be unduly challenging in terms of the degree of change sought. Nevertheless while the focus at the "stability" end of the continuum will be on social support through community care networks, or enabling advice and information services, for example, work in these quadrants can lead to more change-oriented community development. Self-help becomes mutual support which can lead to skill development through various forms of community education, and thus to increased self-esteem, and raised awareness of the potential for collective work for change. This can be the precursor for setting up cooperatives or

FIGURE 1. The Four-Square Model of Community Practice

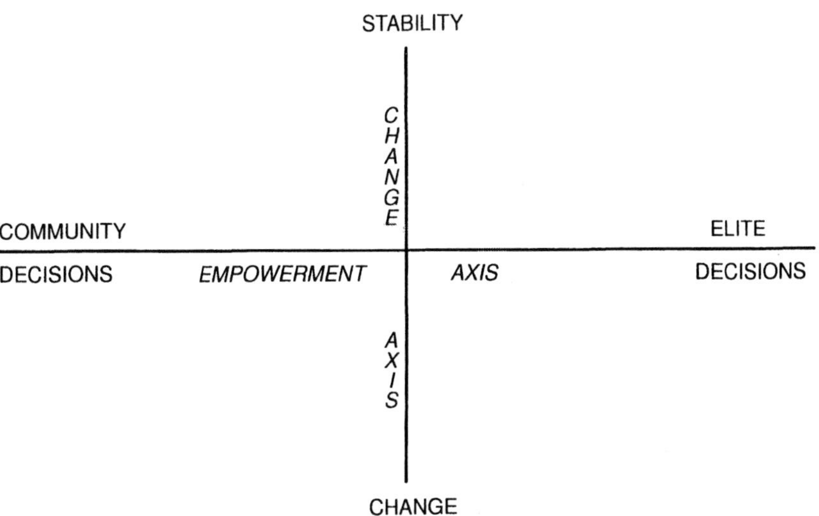

community managed or owned services, centres, businesses with the support of, or in partnership with, local departments, agencies, and business organisations and to community economic development. It can also lead to the development of independent community organisations.

With regard to the horizontal axis, work that originates in or is intended to facilitate the empowerment and thus the involvement of community members in decision making and which either has broad societal support or does not rock the apple cart, would fit into quadrant A. On the other hand in quadrant B one can envision work that stresses the provision and co-ordination of services by local authorities or by bodies designated and/or supported by them, i.e., elite led–the sort of thing Rothman was referring to under his Social Planning model. However, work in this quadrant can range along the horizontal continuum with, at one end, little stress on the involvement of community people, to Local Authority Departments planning and operating services in collaboration with a range of organisations from the voluntary and private sector and increasingly, as one moves along the continuum, with the participation of community members and group representatives.

Rothman's Models A and B, Community Development and Social Planning, thus could be said to fit into quadrants A and B. His Model C, Social Action, is definitely more partisan and confrontational, which is consistent with the more change-oriented and community decision-making ends of each axis, i.e., quadrant C. Under Social Action Rothman saw the stress on direct action by oppressed communities aimed at coercing change from reluctant elites. Hence it would fit at the community decision making end of the empowerment continuum and the change end of the vertical continuum. Workers funded by Local Authority Departments or related agencies would not be expected to last long in post if this became a dominant mode of operation!

Closely aligned with Model C Rothman initially suggested (1970, p. 34) the possibility of another change-oriented model which stressed collaboration between expert leaders of social action organisations with similar interests. They would build as wide a coalition as possible to press for change at a societal level. These leaders are elites in that they form a steering group to make decisions on behalf of the wider membership and assume responsibility for orchestrating regional and national campaigns often aimed at legislative change. Like Stinson, I have found it pertinent to flesh out and incorporate Rothman's Social Reform idea into the four-square schema as Model D. As this work also involves efforts to identify sympathetic office holders in the ruling power structures to help promote the cause, Model D fits appropriately in the four-square framework next to Model C and beneath Model B. It is at the change end of the continuum and also at the elite decision-making end.

This then is how I presented Rothman's Models to students for many years (even as I was seeking to refine it to better reflect practice developments in the U.K.). (See Figure 2.)

Before proceeding to consider how well this model has stood the test of time and its applicability beyond North America, perhaps it would help to consider how well it meets the criteria developed earlier for an analytic model, namely: to abstract essential elements from complex situations, to predict outcomes of actions, to plan

FIGURE 2. Four Basic Modes of Community Practice

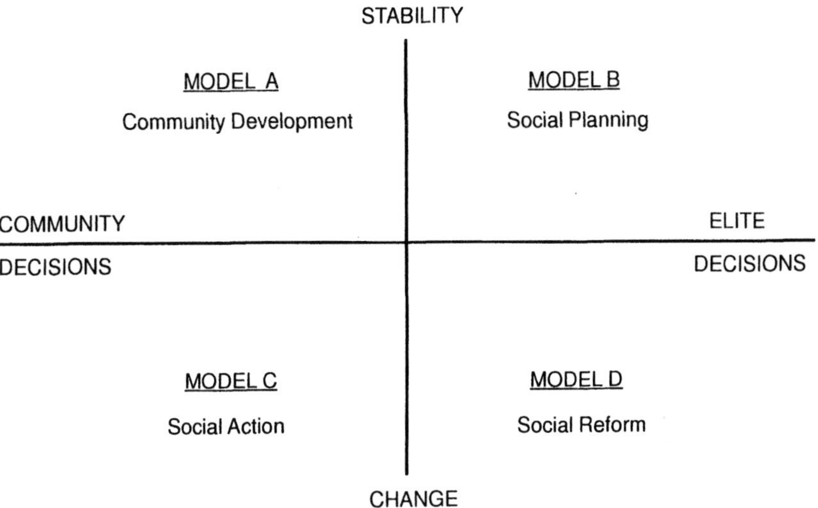

accordingly. A personal example of my introduction to Rothman's modelling approach will illustrate its utility in my experience at least.

CASE STUDY

When James Foreman promulgated his Doctrine of Reparations in the late 1960s he urged that it be taken up by Black activists across the United States. (Here the action starts in quadrant D.) The local Black Economic Development League in Ann Arbor, Michigan did just this, joining forces with an active Welfare Rights Organisation to take dramatic, non-violent, direct action (quadrant C). They began to walk into churches during the Sunday Service and take over the pulpit to read the Doctrine of Reparations. Horrified congregations turned to the courts to get orders banning BEDL/WRO members from local churches and synogues! As young members of a small church, in an integrated part of the city, with a commitment to social action we were horrified likewise at this reaction. We had been working with the WRO women to facilitate their use of our church building as a drop-in centre. What could we do now? A meeting was held with Jack Rothman who at that time was a professor at the University of Michigan.

Professor Rothman introduced us to his modelling work. Applying his approach to this situation we could both comprehend what BEDL/WRO were trying to achieve, why they had to do it in this way, and what we could expect once their organisation and their situation were taken seriously. Understanding this we could see what we needed to do as members of the white congregations who by now had formed a Coalition of Congregations to deal with this perceived threat. Two of us ran for election onto the Executive Committee of this Coalition with the aim of educating the membership about the level of poverty and the social and racial injustices in our community. Based on our study of poverty in the county, our working party was asked to prepare a report for the Governor of Michigan. Poverty and Race Awareness Teach-ins were arranged for the Coalition. Executive Members went out to meet with a variety of community leaders.

This was a very tense time in the community with rumours of 'hit lists' and fear of Detroit City type riots abounding. We risked being written off as part of the white racist oppressive society. Being clear about what we were doing and why was essential. Thanks to the credibility we had established with members of the WRO, we were able to meet secretly with the BEDL leadership to try to explain and discuss our actions and eventually to pave the way for formal meetings. Just as Rothman had predicted, once attitudes in the Coalition changed we moved into a negotiation phase with BEDL/WRO. Eventually the Coalition became a major money raising source for community groups across the community, including for BEDL/WRO (quadrants A & B). Two of the Neighborhood Centres established at that time were still in operation the last time I visited Ann Arbor in the early 1990s. For us the models clearly had analytic and predictive value.

APPLICATION OF THE FOUR-SQUARE MODELLING FRAME TO THE U.K.

What about the applicability of the model in the United Kingdom? While the variables still seem to be the crucial ones in terms of analysis, *the first problem* I had in applying Rothman's Models to community work in the U.K. was that the Social Planning Mode really did not seem to fit so well with the British Community Work situation. Here Social Work is distinct from Community Work. Practitioners follow different routes to unique qualifications, whilst in the U.S.A. Community Organisation is a form of Social Work. Although there has always been a dedicated cadre of social workers in the U.K. who see the importance of Community Social Work (Hadley, Cooper, Dale, & Stacey, 1990), Community Workers traditionally would be horrified to be called Social Workers and would rarely see themselves as having a Social Planning orientation in the way modelled by Rothman. While Thomas and Twelvetrees, for example, distinguish between Professional and Socialist Schools within British Community Work, the Professional School still would be more associated with Locality/Community Development and the Socialist School with Social Action. Although the Professional School would recognise the importance of liaison with Social Planners as part of their community organisation work, after the demise of the CD Projects (see Popple, this volume) they would rarely have been employed by them.

From a study undertaken in 1991 on community development in Plymouth (Lewis, Jeffries, & Levitt) it was clear, however, that Local Authority Departments actually were the sponsors in one form or another of the bulk of community development work being undertaken in the area at that time. Indeed our study itself had been commissioned by an inter-agency coalition. It is interesting to note that Rothman (this volume) makes a similar point in his discussion of Locality Development–External Linkages, noting that "A dilemma is that often locality development programs are sponsored and funded by outside entities."

This vividly illustrated how community workers were inevitably involved to some degree with social planning or with those responsible for the provision or purchase of health, housing, social, education or leisure services and increasingly in promoting community economic development. As part of this study I also conducted a review of community development in 15 different local authority areas in England and Wales which revealed (Lewis, Jeffries, & Levitt, p. 11):

> *a widely held commitment to integrated strategies for community development within regions or areas which can help to: (a) secure funding; (b) develop human resources; (c) share good practice; (d) create partnerships across organisational boundaries and between organisations and communities; (e) facilitate training.*
>
> *The first priority is to break with the service* ***delivery*** *mentality, focusing instead on planning* ***with*** *the community in order to enable the community to act for itself.*

In terms of Model B therefore it seems more pertinent to recast this as Partnership Promotion (PP). Indeed effective Community Development clearly is facilitated by collaboration between aware and sensitive public, private and voluntary organisations committed to Community Development, and active community groups whose members can hold their own in such partnership situations. Thus, from the community point of view, to be a partner in community development implies community groups composed of people with an awareness of what is needed and the confidence to contribute to community development strategies. Partnership Promotion of Community Development can be a natural progression from efforts by departments and agencies to build supportive and informed community networks at the stability end of the change continuum. Efforts to promote community management of services or community economic development can be envisaged at the lower end of the change axis in the upper quadrants. However it is important to bear in mind that this also will need to be underpinned by considerable work in supporting and promoting the capacity of community members to maintain involvement at this level of community organisation. For this sort of collaborative community development, skills to negotiate, advocate, mediate and contract also become very important. Community groups need to be able to apply for and handle funds, participate in and run meetings, write reports, and organise publicity.

In short, when closely analysed it becomes apparent that much of the work in quadrant A is about developing or giving scope for and recognition to the skills, or capacities, of community groups. Thus work in this quadrant could more accurately be described as Capacity and Awareness Promotion (CAP). (I use the term 'promotion' advisedly as for me it has a more empowering connotation than 'building,' i.e, the ability is there, it just needs to be given a chance to blossom.) On the other hand, much of the work in quadrant B could be about what Weil and Gamble refer to as *"making social planning more accessible and inclusive in a community, to connect social and economic investments to grassroots groups, to advocate for broad coalitions in solving community problems, and to infuse the social planning process with a concern for social justice" (p. 580).* This means that Community Development (CD) itself is in reality the outcome of work in the two quadrants A and B (see Figure 3).

The *second problem* with the model was that the separation of Community Development/Capacity Promotion from Social Action did not make clear that the former is also vital for the latter. Community Workers in Britain from the Socialist School tended to dismiss Capacity and Awareness Promotion (CAP) work as 'social work' stressing the collective nature of community work. This struck me as somewhat ironic when you consider the role of the Worker's Education Association in the Labour Movement. In fact most community workers do spend a lot of time in face to face work before they can coalesce interests into action groups. Interpersonal, educational and group work skills seemed to be under-developed in the training of British Community Workers. Both feminist analysis and practice and the work of Paulo Freire (1981) make clear the importance, in terms of situations that are going to require more dramatic action to achieve change, of starting with the personal concerns of community people–'starting where people are' as Freire puts it.

FIGURE 3. Collaborative Community Development: Two Quadrants

Collaborative Community Development

Quadrant A	Quadrant B
Capacity & Awareness Promotion CAP	Partnership Promotion PP

Organisations of various oppressed peoples, such as Black activists in the U.S. Civil Rights Movement, also realised and demonstrated the power of linking opportunities for skill development (such as literacy skills necessary for voter registration) with awareness raising as to the possibilities and legitimacy of direct action for change. Thus the Declaration of Independence becomes a text for learning to read (Jeffries, 1994, p. 129).

In short the model needed to suggest the relationship between raising awareness and capacity building and more radical change-oriented work. CAP can be a precursor for change-oriented protest or Nonviolent Direct Action (NDA) as well as for Collaborative Community Development. Obviously collective non-violent direct action is unlikely to be sustained unless considerable organisation and skill building work has been undertaken first, as Rothman stressed (1970, p. 26).

Thus when initial analysis using the four fundamental variables suggested earlier (p. 4) has indicated that the worker is involved with an oppressed or disenfranchised community, considerable change is suggested. It is also unlikely that there will be much readiness to engage in CCD. The community needs to get the attention of those in authority but first they must develop the conviction and the confidence for such bold community organising. Action aimed at gaining the attention of an unsympathetic power structure will need to be underpinned by CAP.

Thus I see sustained Social Action being bimodal in that it bridges quadrants A and C. Envisioning an outer ring of bimodal bridging approaches points to the fact that it is quite possible for communities basically pursuing an overall CCD approach to utilise NDA tactics to, for example, galvanise support in their community or to renew the commitment of CCD partners to working *with* the community group. Thus we see a two-tier model developing, the outer ring of which makes clear what sort of mixing and phasing strategies are likely to be most compatible with the inner, core mode initially chosen. It is good to read that this is very much in tune with the phasing and mixing refinements Rothman has now developed. The four-square frame, with its bridging outer ring is perhaps a less complicated, if less sophisticated, way to model this as a developmental process. (See Figure 4.)

FIGURE 4. Collaborative Community Development: Three Quadrants

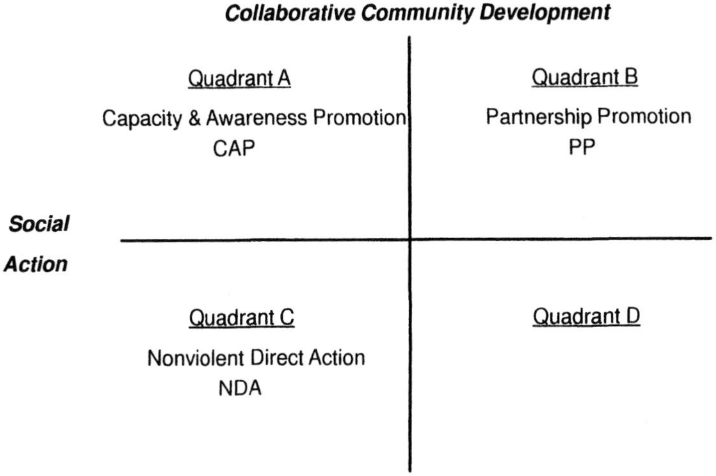

Collaborative Community Development

	Quadrant A Capacity & Awareness Promotion CAP	Quadrant B Partnership Promotion PP
Social Action		
	Quadrant C Nonviolent Direct Action NDA	Quadrant D

This leaves us with a *third issue:* how to model the campaign/coalition building work that we labelled Mode D and on which Rothman puts much more stress in his latest work. Clearly social campaigns have long been a key feature not only of single issue organising but also of radical, change-oriented social movements. While the former often have a more specific objective and may align themselves with organisational elites, the latter are more comprehensive in scope. They may be seeking social justice or be promoting an ecological consciousness in society. Just as NDA is a vital part of Social Action so it is also seen as an essential aspect of social movements. But NDA alone would not be enough. These days campaign organisers can take advantage of information technology to build country-wide and international campaign coalitions. Yet to generate the mass mobilisation that may be necessary to take on multi-nationals or an unsympathetic government, it is important also to have strong community level organisation.

I had concluded that Rothman's Three Modes did not adequately model this interface. However if quadrant C is typified by the use of Nonviolent Direct Action, often as a part of Social Action, and quadrant D by building Social Campaigning Coalitions, Mass

Social Movements clearly combine these approaches. Social Movements, which obviously fit at the extreme end of the change continuum, thus can be seen to bridge quadrants C and D. This last bimodal approach would come into its own when large segments of the populations feel that they are being ignored by the standard democratic processes and that their rights are consistently repressed.

By including social campaigning as the fourth mode the four-square frame resolves the problem Rothman alludes to in his latest work on models, namely that Social Action "has two essentially different types of goals–'radical change goals' that aim at fundamental alterations in society; and 'reformist goals' that aim at incremental alterations, which in turn rely on collaboration between elites at certain stages in the process" (Rothman, this volume, p. 90). Clearly, once specific Social Campaigns are taken seriously enough by those with policy planning and decision making power, attention should turn again to negotiation (as Rothman stressed in regard to Social Action) in the hopes of achieving Social Reform. From this there is potential to move on to demand a more inclusive approach to Social Planning and thus back to Collaborative Community Development. Thus Social Planning and Reform can be presented as the fourth bimodal combination, nicely squaring the outer circle. A case study from the U.K. follows in order to illustrate the mixing and phasing of the central core modes of practice and the outer bridging modes. (See Figure 5.)

PEMBROKE STREET ESTATE MANAGEMENT BOARD

Work by the Devon Cooperative Development Agency (D.C.D.A.) with council housing residents and the Plymouth City Housing Department illustrates the way both quadrant A and B modes are required for collaborative community development and how this can be prompted by developments in Social Planning or Social Action.

The physical deterioration of their locality and the perceived reluctance of the local Housing Department to address their concerns adequately, led some tenants of this very deprived area to contact the D.C.D.A. in 1989. The tenants who were active in the Pembroke Street Residents Association opted to push for a full-blown management co-operative to run their estate instead of the

FIGURE 5. The Four-Square Modeling Frame

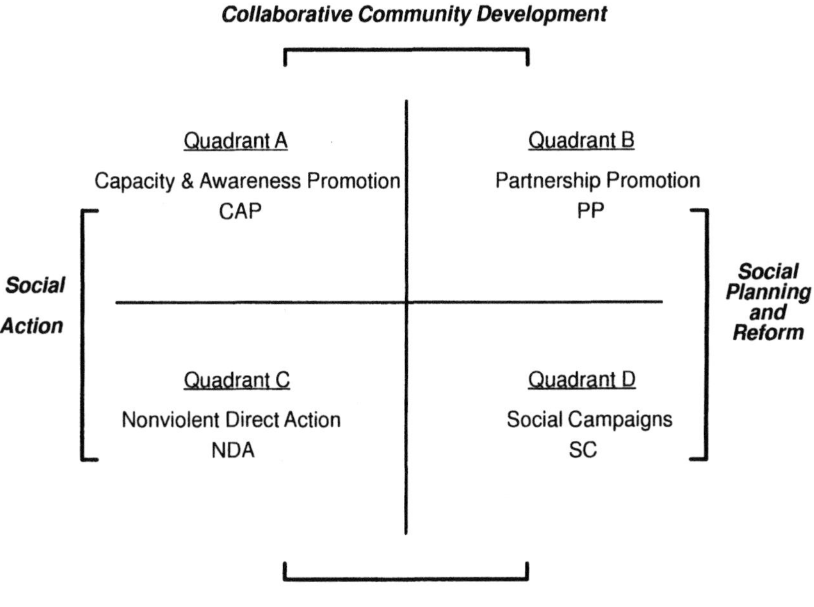

Housing Department. However, despite apparent support, as indicated in a canvas of all tenants, uncertainty as to the practical effects of such a radical change led to a split in the community.

Deep-seated divisions were magnified in the climate of uncertainty about the future of public housing as a consequence of the Conservative government's moves to privatise public housing in Britain. An alternative residents' group emerged in favour of the estate management remaining with the Housing Department. Eventually a way forward was found which was acceptable to both groups and DCDA workers could proceed in a manner synonymous with the Capacity and Awareness Promotion mode. In the meantime work had been underway also in paving the way for Partnership Promotion (quadrant B). Good relations had been established with the Housing Department Officers, which was crucial in terms of their willingness to collaborate in this innovative proposal.

The initial focus was on the immediate concerns of residents. DCDA helped tenants negotiate both with the Housing Department to rent a unit as a community flat, and with the Social Services Department for money for the first year's rent. In the process residents developed important skills that could be built upon in later stages of the work. They also began to establish credibility with key decision-makers, as well as demonstrating to other residents that changes could be made. The Community Flat proved a great success being used by a variety of groups of all ages. The DCDA ran training sessions there. Some of these were directly related to preparing for tenant management (such as IT and committee skills); others were spin-offs, such as a basic business familiarisation course for a small group of women.

The plan that was negotiated to the satisfaction of both groups of residents proposed tenant management of the estate in partnership with the Local Authority. The new Housing Act perhaps had the unanticipated effect of prompting a partnership ethos within the Housing Department because of concerns that if given the choice, as was possible under the new legislation, if they were too disgruntled tenants would opt to have their estates run by private companies. Thus we see Social Planning at the macro level promoting Mode B action at the micro level.

It was agreed that the thirteen residents on the Board would have responsibility for prioritising expenditure of the £90,000 annual budget on matters such as security, landscaping, caretaking and repairs. The City Council would continue to set rent levels and have responsibility for collecting the rent. A district wide Estate Management Action Strategy was developed. This involved cost benefit analysis and a comprehensive bid for refurbishment of the whole area to the tune of £6.25 million. The hope was that this would cover not only extensive refurbishment and upgrading of the properties and immediate environs but also the building of a Community Centre.

The outcome has been an integrated training, employment and refurbishment programme. In addition to those employed as a result of the initial tenant management co-op, a few residents set up a cleaning and a security co-op. Many more participated in the Pembroke Street community architecture scheme, with residents involved in designs for the external appearance of the buildings, landscaping and railings. Other economic and crime prevention initiatives in the general area have followed. The demolition and redevelopment of poor quality adjacent housing has also begun.

This is a classic example of collaborative community development requiring co-operation between community groups and a wide variety of agencies such as the City Housing Department, Inner Area Programme, City Estates, Department of Employment, Police and so on. D.C.D.A. acted as a catalyst in this process, taking advantage of their contacts and credibility to intervene at the right point in the policy making process to promote partnerships and ensure that policies and initiatives facilitate grassroot development projects. As a result changes have been made which will benefit residents in other low-income areas of the city. For example it was decided to set up a job skills register so that local people could be called upon to apply for jobs generated as part of the refurbishment of the estate. For this to be realistic union concerns had to be addressed and means found to ensure that contractors did give preference to those listed on the local skills register.

This also illustrates the potential for professionally trained development workers, who understand the policy-making process, to act as brokers between the community and local policy makers. It illustrates the need, if one has any hope of generating significant change from the grassroots, for community workers to find a way to promote partnerships. In Plymouth a key part of the Co-operative Development Agency's work has been to cultivate contacts with agencies such as Task Force Plymouth, Plymouth Development Corp., Devon and Cornwall TEC, the City's own Employment and Economy Committee, etc. This illustrates how collaborative community economic development which is grounded in the local community can contribute to change in economic and service structures at the local level and potentially even at the national level. Thus micro level work in quadrants A and B can itself influence macro level Social Planning. For example, D.C.D.A. is convinced that publicity relating to the development of the Pembroke Street Cooperative Estate Management Board had a part in the national 1994 "Right To Manage" legislation.

With due regard to the ongoing need to promote group work

skills, a ripple effect can result which provides a base of good will and a more positive foundation upon which to start other revitalization activities. That this can happen in a period of deep recession, and in areas renowned for their entrenched problems, is perhaps the most significant testimony for the empowering potential of promoting both a partnership orientation in local government and the capacity of residents.

The key variable is perhaps the nature of the partnership involved in the particular project. If the various economic development stakeholders are committed to *partnership with* the community, they will appreciate the multi-dimensionality of collaborative community development. When so much depends on the motivation, commitment and skills of the co-operators, there can be no short cuts. The interests and strengths of people in the community have to be recognised, developed and supported at each stage of the process. This means that there must be careful collaboration and educative work with local government officers as well as in the community to ensure funding for both the early stages, and ongoing maintenance support aspects, of the work.

THE RELATIONSHIP OF THE FOUR-SQUARE MODEL TO OTHER PAPERS IN THIS VOLUME

To test the four-square model let us consider how it relates to the Weil and Gamble Table of Models reprinted in this volume. While some of their comparative characteristics relate to what I have suggested is the second stage of analysis, namely to determining strategies, roles and methods (and Weil/Gamble provide more specificity than Rothman as to change target, scope and beneficiaries), it is clear from the variables indicated which of the four-square quadrants relate to which of the Weil/Gamble models. Furthermore, it captures the most likely ways in which, as Rothman points out (this volume): "intervention approaches overlap and are used in mixed form in practice."

It is important to note that Weil and Gamble differentiate between geographic communities (their Model One) and Functional (or interest) Communities (Model Two). In Britain we are used to using the term 'community' to hold various forms of social association. While the Weil/Gamble distinction is useful for the second level of action planning, it is clear that from the point of view of initial analysis both have a focus on capacity and awareness building. Indeed the Weil/Gamble Models One, Two, Three, and Five would all seem to be aspects of Collaborative Community Development, with One and Three focusing more on CAP, though at different points in regard to both the change and empowerment continuum. Model Two could involve work also in either quadrant C or B; Model Four in B and perhaps D and Six would be situated in the lower quadrants. Model Seven has more stress on Social Action with CAP work implied as well as the possibility of direct action.

The Weil/Gamble Model Eight obviously is an example of the way social movements bridge quadrants C and D, moving the Social Action mode of 'Functional Community Organising' into comprehensive Social Movements, such as the Women's Movement. Here grassroots local level Non-violent Direct Action coincides with nationwide political campaigning aimed at legislative and/or service and organisational reform. The vision is nothing less than the transformation of society and the way we work together, whether in agencies or coalitions or partnerships or grassroot community groups. This could be envisioned as a circle at the intersection of the four quadrants and illustrates that feminist organising is far more comprehensive and sophisticated than bimodal social action, as Rothman implies in his Figure 1.4 in this volume.

The following figure is an attempt to more explicitly relate the four-square model to the modes of practice suggested by Weil and Gamble and by Popple. It should be remembered that the vertical axis starts at the top with supportive work and moves down towards the more change oriented community economic development mode, to Public Advocacy, Coalition Building. When the mode title straddles on the vertical line this is to suggest the work actively encourages partnership. When the mode has been placed over to the right in quadrant B or D it indicates that the decision-making involves elites; when it is in quadrant A or C it means that the community is involved in decision making. (See Figure 6.)

In short the Weil/Gamble modes of practice would seem to be complementary to the modelling frame proposed in this paper. I would suggest a practitioner on both sides of the Atlantic could first

FIGURE 6. The Four-Square Modeling Frame Related to Modes of Practice

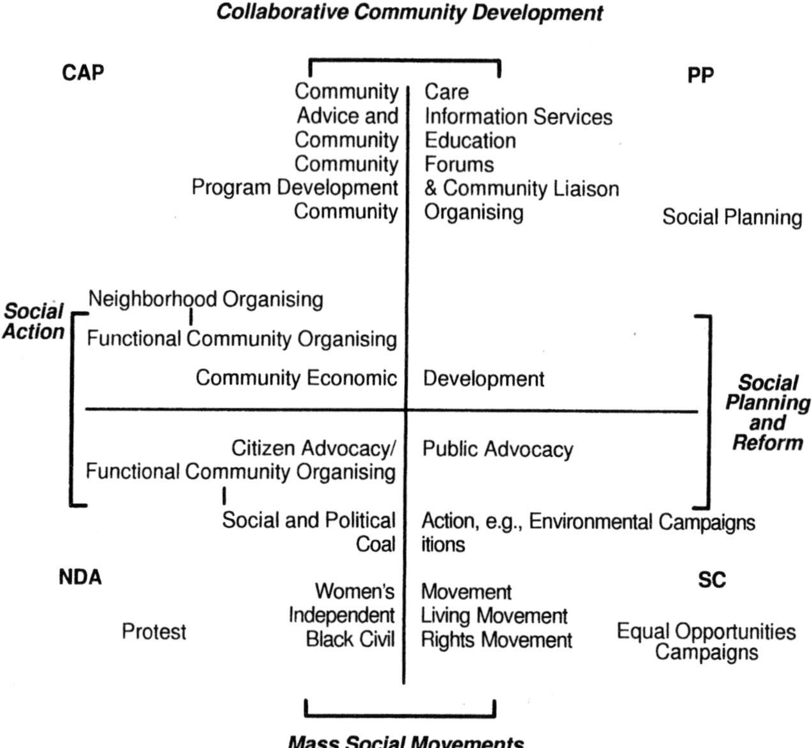

use the four-square model to gain their basic orientation and then look in more depth at examples of modes that fit that fundamental orientation and reflect their cultural context. The latter will help the practitioner to clarify objectives, strategies and tactics that could fit their particular circumstances.

In conclusion, it is my contention that this refined four-square model, with its outer bimodal bridging approaches, not only provides a simple analytic model that a community practitioner can use to help make sense of our rapidly changing social and political environment and assess the likely outcomes of pursuing various approaches, but that it also encapsulates the way these approaches relate to and build upon each other in practice.

NOTE

1. I was first introduced to the use of the four-square framework for presenting Rothman's 'Models' in a lecture by Professor Arthur Stinson, formerly from the School of Social Work at Carleton University, Ottawa, Canada. As far as I know he never published this. Over the years I have significantly modified his basic idea, as I will develop in this paper.

REFERENCES

Checkoway, B. (1995). Six strategies of community change. *Community Development Journal*, 30(1), 2-20.

Freire, P. (1981). *Pedagogy of the Oppressed*. New York: Continuum Press.

Hadley, R., Cooper, M., Dale, P., & Stacey, G. (1990). *A community social worker's handbook*. Tavistock Publications.

Lewis, J., Jeffries, A., Levitt, I. (1991). Report on *Developing an Approach to Community Development in Plymouth*, Plymouth, UK: Polytechnic South West.

Jeffries, A. (1994). Coalescing a variety of discourses: Community organising in the United States. In S. Jacobs and K. Popple (Eds.). *Community work in the 1990s*. Nottingham: Spokesman.

Popple, K. (1995). *Analysing community work: Its theory and practice*. Buckingham-Philadelphia: Open University Press.

Popple, K. (1996). Community Work: British Models. *Journal of Community Practice*, 3(3/4), 147-179.

Rothman, J. (1970). Three models of community organisation. In F. Cox, J. Erlich, J. Rothman & J. Tropman (Eds.). *Strategies of community organisation*. Itaska, IL: Peacock Publishing.

Rothman, J. (1995). Approaches to community intervention. In *Strategies of community intervention* (Fifth Edition). J. Rothman, J. L. Erlich, J. E. Tropman, with F. Cox (Eds.). Itaska, IL: F.E. Peacock Publishers, Inc.

Rothman, J. (1996). The Interweaving of Community Intervention Approaches. *Journal of Community Practice*, 3(3/4), 69-99.

Thomas, D. N. (1983). *The making of community work*. London: George Allen & Unwin.

Twelvetrees, A. (1991). *Community work* (2nd ed.). London: Macmillan.

Weil, M. O., & Gamble, D. N. (1995). Community Practice Models. In *Encyclopedia of Social Work* (19th ed.) (pp. 577-593). Washington, DC: NASW.

A Feminist Response to Rothman's "The Interweaving of Community Intervention Approaches"

Cheryl Hyde, PhD

SUMMARY. This paper critiques Jack Rothman's "The Interweaving of Community Intervention Approaches" (this volume) from a feminist perspective. A feminist version of his intervention typology, using a wide range of exemplars, is constructed. It suggests the scope of feminism not recognized in his account. Discussion centers on the construction of this feminist typology, which illuminates problems inherent in a categorical approach to community practice, such as Rothman's. It is argued that much would be gained by recognizing the dimensions of ideology, longitudinal development, and commitment within community intervention and incorporating social movement literature into practice analyses. *[Article copies available for a fee from The Haworth Document Delivery Service: 1-800-342-9678. E-mail address: getinfo@ haworth.com]*

KEYWORDS. Feminist organizing, community intervention, macro practice

One of the first articles read by this author as an incoming MSW student was Jack Rothman's "Three Models of Community Orga-

---

Cheryl Hyde is Assistant Professor of Social Work at Boston University.

Address correspondence to: Cheryl Hyde, Assistant Professor, School of Social Work, Boston University, 264 Bay State Road, Boston, MA 02215.

The author thanks Marie Weil and the anonymous reviewers for their suggestions.

[Haworth co-indexing entry note]: "A Feminist Response to Rothman's 'The Interweaving of Community Intervention Approaches.'" Hyde, Cheryl. Co-published simultaneously in *Journal of Community Practice* (The Haworth Press, Inc.) Vol. 3, No. 3/4, 1996, pp. 127-145; and: *Community Practice: Conceptual Models* (ed: Marie Weil) The Haworth Press, Inc., 1996, pp. 127-145. Single or multiple copies of this article are available for a fee from The Haworth Document Delivery Service [1-800-342-9678, 9:00 a.m. - 5:00 p.m. (EST). E-mail address: getinfo@haworth.com].

nization Practice, Their Mixing and Phasing" (1979).[1] It was a rather straightforward attempt to categorize different forms of community practice. Yet in some ways, it failed to satisfy many macro practitioners because Rothman had not fully tapped the richness or complexity of community based work; apparently a conclusion he has also reached. In his most recent version, included in this volume, Rothman seeks to refine, update, expand, and reformulate his earlier work. It is a wide-ranging and impressive effort.

This decision to "try to tidy things up" (Rothman, 1995, p. 26) is largely grounded in attempting to incorporate myriad ways, some representing new innovations since the earlier publication, that community practitioners go about their craft. One important development within the community practice literature was that feminist perspectives on organizing finally received overdue recognition (Brandwein, 1981; Gutierrez & Lewis, 1992; Hyde, 1989; Weil, 1986). To Rothman's credit, he appreciates and includes feminist examples in his revision.

The purpose of this essay is to examine and critique Rothman's use of these feminist cases, and in doing so, raise larger analytical issues for those who are "students of community practice" to consider. First, Rothman's understanding of feminist approaches to community intervention, as well as his designation of feminist endeavors in his three core models, are summarized. As a partially corrective measure to his treatment of feminism, feminist examples for all his intervention modes and mixes are then offered. The paper concludes with a discussion of concerns with respect to Rothman's use of feminist organizing and of lessons learned from delineating feminist forms for all community interventions. Specifically, arguments are made for the import of ideology, longer term development, and commitment in community intervention models, for greater clarity with respect to what is meant by community and whether certain community types foster particular intervention modes, and finally, for the incorporation of insights from social movement literature into practice analyses. These concerns are not limited to Rothman's work, but are challenges to the broader field.

Before proceeding, however, it is necessary to clarify the difference between feminist and women's organizing. Often used interchangeably, in this paper they are not. Feminism is:

> . . . minimally the recognition that women, compared to men, are an oppressed group and that women's problems are a result of discrimination. . . . . Feminism's political perspective is pro-woman and favors changes to improve women's collective status, living conditions, opportunities, power, and self-esteem. A feminist organization, therefore, is pro-woman, political and socially transformational. (Martin, 1990, p. 184)

Feminist organizing, therefore, is about changing power structures and processes in order to achieve gender equity. Both men and women (at least in this author's view) may be beneficiaries or supporters of feminist endeavors. In contrast, women's organizing does not necessarily embrace the goals of feminism (though it might). For example, right wing leader Phyllis Schlafly has organized a woman's group called the Eagle Forum. Its purpose is to maintain and enhance traditional gender roles. She does women's organizing, yet it certainly is not feminist. Female composition, alone, does not make either an organization or change effort feminist; ideologies, goals, and desired outcomes that challenge gender-based oppression, do (Hyde, 1989, 1992, 1995a; Ferree & Martin, 1995a).

THE THREE MODELS AND FEMINISM

Rothman (1979) identified three models or ideal types of community intervention: social action, locality development, and social planning. He then suggested that these models may be combined into action/development, action/planning, and planning/development. In the latest version, Rothman (this volume) further elaborates by suggesting that one model in a combination could dominate the other. For example, one could have action/development as balanced, favoring action, or favoring development characteristics. Rothman's highly illustrative Figure 1.5, "The Paradigm of Community Intervention Showing Examples of Organizational Types for Each Mode of Intervention and Mixed Forms" (p. 81), captures the range of possibilities by linking organizational illustrations to intervention approach.

Rothman cites feminist examples with respect to locality development, social action, and the balanced action/development categories. Locality development is a "community building endeavor" that fosters community competency and integration. It is inherently self-help in orientation. There is an assumption that the contesting groups will be able to reconcile their differences; thus, communication and consensus skills are stressed. Rothman notes the overlap between this mode and feminist approaches to organizing because both emphasize "wide participation, concern for democratic procedure and educational goals–including consciousness raising" (1995, p. 29).

Social action "aims at making fundamental changes in the community, including the redistribution of power and resources and gaining access to decision-making for marginal groups" (1995, p. 32). Within this mode, there is a "militant orientation" in which confrontational or adversarial strategies are employed to legitimate the grievances of and secure benefits for disenfranchised people. Rothman includes feminist organizing groups in a long list of action organizations (e.g., ACORN, United Farm Workers). He also suggests that feminist organizing, epitomized by the slogan "the personal is political," exemplifies those social action groups that embrace process goals, especially constituency development (1995, p. 36).

Feminist organizing is also cited as an exemplar of the balanced form of the development/action combination. Paraphrasing aspects of this author's work on macro feminist practice (Hyde, 1989), Rothman asserts:

> . . . that feminist organizing comprises a combination of traits that are traditionally considered feminine with those that are often considered masculine. The feminine aspect includes humanistic qualities such as caring and nurturance, coupled with use of democratic processes and structures. . . . These aspects are all associated with the locality development mode.
>
> At the same time, the feminist organizing perspective is concerned with fundamental cultural and political change–the elimination of patriarchy. . . . These tougher, more militant elements of practice in the past often have been associated with a masculine posture and the social action intervention mode. (this volume, pp. 78-79)

Setting aside for the moment whether this gendered notion of revolution is an accurate one (it is not), Rothman clearly argues that a feminist organizing perspective "is a balanced composite of practice variables involving assumptions and goals of social action joined with those involving the methods of locality development" (this volume, p. 79).

Interestingly, Rothman offers no feminist illustrations for the social planning and policy approach, a "technical process of problem-solving regarding substantive social problems" (1995, p. 30), or for the various action/planning and planning/development mixtures. It is not clear, however, if this is due to an inability to find existing examples or to the belief that because planning and policy is a rational process involving the "assembling and analyzing [of] data to prescribe means for solving social problems" (1995, p. 30), it is somehow antithetical to feminist principles.

FEMINIST EXAMPLES OF COMMUNITY INTERVENTION

While the inclusion of feminist approaches to community practice is welcomed, problems nonetheless exist with Rothman's interpretation and use of intervention models. The origin of this critique is situated in Figure 1.5 (this volume, p. 81). In this diagram, which is reinforced by much of the text, Rothman uses organizations to signify intervention modes, with one exception. The balanced development/action combination is illustrated by feminist organiz*ing*. The disagreement is not that some feminist organizing endeavors exhibit the characteristics of the development/action approach. Rather, the problem is that a political perspective, "feminist," and a process, "organizing," are mistakenly equated with "organization," a formal (more or less) structure that serves as a vehicle through which mobilization can occur.

This designation suggests a lack of clarity as to what the unit of analysis is or ought to be (addressed later in the discussion). It also clouds a comprehensive understanding of feminist endeavors. Rothman, perhaps unintentionally, reinforces a monolithic notion of feminism, as in "the feminist perspective," rather than understanding that many feminisms exist. Feminist intervention projects can be found across all of Rothman's modes (singular and combined) because the many faces of feminist ideology transcend various organizational types and intervention modes.

In order to demonstrate the complexity and scope of feminist enterprises and lay the foundation for a broader discussion of Rothman's overall approach to community intervention, his Figure 1.5 is recreated with only feminist illustrations. All organizational examples are guided either explicitly or implicitly by basic feminist principles including the centrality of relationships; consciousness raising; reconceptualization of power; democratizing processes and structures; and fundamental cultural and structural change (Hyde, 1989). Some are revolutionary and some are reform in orientation; all originate in the second wave of feminism which "officially" emerged in the 1960s and continues today. For the most part lesser known projects, as opposed to the more famous ones such as the National Organization for Women, are highlighted. The sample also reflects the diversity within the movement. Table 1 conveys some feminist illustrations for each intervention.

First, consider the "pure" models: social action, locality development and social planning. There is an endless list of feminist social action organizations. Several such groups were formed near the end of the ERA ratification drive, including the Congressional Union (Elam, 1989) and Women Rising in Resistance (Sargent, 1989). Both employed militant and confrontational strategies, such as hunger strikes and civil disobedience, to press for the passage of this amendment. Contrary to assertions that the current feminist movement is dead or dormant, many action organizations were founded in recent years. One example is the Lesbian Avengers, heir to the radical, guerilla theater techniques of the women's liberation movement of the late 1960s and early 1970s. Lesbian Avengers stage typically provocative protests on behalf of women, gays and lesbians, and other oppressed groups, concluding these public demonstrations with displays of fire eating. Many current forms of feminist protest groups use culturally oriented tactics, such as art or music, as part of their strategic repertoire.

There also are many examples of locality development. As Rothman correctly notes, there is a clear connection between this modality's emphasis on self-help and feminist endeavors. Many anti-violence and health centers, which emphasize service and education, fit

TABLE 1. Community Interventions, Organizational Types, and Feminist Examples

Community Interventions	Organizational Types	Feminist Examples
Social Action	Green Peace	Congressional Union Lesbian Avengers
Action+/ Development	Farm Workers Union	Chicago Women's Liberation Union Nine to Five
Action/ Development	Feminist Organizing	Vimochana Project Oasis
Action/ Development+	Neighborhood Block Clubs	Greenham Peace Camp Coal. for Women's Safety
Locality Development	Peace Corps	Women's Self Defense Council L.A. Woman's Building
Development+/ Planning	National Ctr for Neighborhood Enterprise	National Council of Neighborhood Women National Institute for Women of Color
Development/ Planning	United Way	Women's Way Emily's List
Development/ Planning+	Citizens Advisory Comm.	PEER Displaced Homemaker Network
Social Planning	Municipal Health Dept.	Institute for Women's Policy Research Femocrats
Planning+/ Action	Governmental Planned Reform	State Commissions on the Status of Women Radcliffe Public Policy Institute
Planning/ Action	Children's Defense Fund	Women's Equity Action League Ct. Women's Educational & Legal Fund
Planning/ Action+	Inst. for Democratic Socialism	Women's Action Coalition Italian League for Divorce

the development category. For example, the Women's Self Defense Council (Searles & Berger, 1987) offered training in self-defense for women from a feminist empowerment perspective (Rothman's "feeling of personal mastery"). Settlement houses also exemplify locality development. Community women's centers, such as the Los Angeles Woman's Building, are feminist versions of the settlement house–" . . . extend[ing] women's culture, sharing it with a large constituency . . . [and] validat[ing] women's actions in the world from a base of mutual support and communitarian values" (de Bretteville, 1980, p. 294). Feminist examples of social planning are more difficult to locate. This may be due to the emphasis on government programs within this category, such as health departments, welfare councils or regional planning groups. Since a feminist government has not yet occurred (except in mythic lore), the options are limited. The Institute for Women's Policy Research, an organization founded to provide relevant research and technical assistance "that contribute[s] to the development of policies and programs that adequately consider women's needs" (Spalter-Roth & Schreiber, 1995, p. 116), captures the essence of the social planning mode. There also are examples of feminist practitioners carving out niches within policy organizations to pursue feminist goals and projects. Weil (1988) documents the efforts within the L.A. County Department of Children's Services Sexual Abuse Program to establish "an alternative program with a collaborative, feminist-oriented organizational subculture" (p. 69). Another case is the "Femocrats," a network of Australian feminist policy-makers who formally coalesced around the need for women-centered reform initiatives (Eisenstein, 1995).

Next, consider the mixed modalities, beginning with action/development categories. As noted above, Rothman asserts that feminist organizing exemplifies the balanced mixture. Indeed, countless organizational and project examples exist, many of which combine service, education, and action. One such case is Vimochana in Bangalore, India, which seeks justice for and protection of women against the practices of wife killings and harassment. Strategies include lobbying, community meetings, and public education campaigns against the often tacitly condoned practices of violence against women ("I cry for help," n.d.). Many battered women's shelters, such as Project Oasis, accomplish similar goals. This organization brings " . . . feminist organizing into multiracial and multiethnic urban communities. The goal of Project Oasis was to end violence against women in these communities through the provisions of advocacy, counseling, and shelter services, and through community education, legal advocacy, and the development of self-help networks" (Gutierrez & Lewis, 1992, p. 122).

Numerous feminist organizations, such as those founded during the heydays of radical feminism, incorporate the mutual aid orientation of the development mode with a strong emphasis on action strategies (action+/development).[2] The Chicago Women's Liberation Union, "an explicitly radical, anti-capitalist, feminist, city-wide organization" ("Statement of purpose: Chicago . . . ", n.d.), was an amalgam of programs with a clear commitment to liberatory mobilization. It housed various direct action projects, such as Women DARE and Action Coalition for Decent Childcare. It also supported various service and education programs, such as the underground abortion collective "Jane" (before the legalization of abortion) and the Women's Liberation School. Even these projects possessed distinct confrontational stances (Strobel, 1995). Union oriented activism also signifies the action+/development approach. Organizations, such as Nine to Five and Coalition of Labor Union Women, sponsor protest and other mobilization efforts, as well as membership development (Ferree & Hess, 1985).

The Peace Encampments, such as those in Puget Sound or Greenham, England (Buehler, 1985; Garland, 1988), are examples that place greater import on development (action/development+). Such efforts seek to create and maintain new, feminist communities of women, yet in doing so, some aspects of the action mode are also present. Simone Wilkinson, a Greenham participant, described her initial involvement in the camp:

> I began getting involved in the camp, and as I spent more time there, my outlook finally began to improve. I had joined the peace movement out of sheer, total despair. . . . Now I was witnessing the creativity of women. They were living on a piece of wasteland, and out of sticks and plastic they had built beautiful shelters. And, what they were doing there was so

> clearcut and simple–just being there, a constant presence, talking to people about their concerns. (Garland, 1988, p. 137)

Another example of this combination is the Coalition for Women's Safety, which is similar, in some ways, to the neighborhood block clubs cited by Rothman. A black, radical feminist organization, the Combahee River Collective, formed this multiracial coalition as a grassroots response to the need for neighborhood safety during a time in which numerous murders of black women in Boston went uninvestigated (Reinharz, 1983).

In Rothman's account, the balanced combination of development and planning is exemplified by the United Way. While not as far-reaching in scope, Women's Way in Philadelphia is a feminist version of the United Way (Brilliant, 1990). It cultivates and funds programs with decidedly feminist orientations. Emily's List, which works within the Democratic Party to identify, advise, and support women's rights candidates, employs planning (technical problem solving) and development (self-help) techniques (Ferree & Martin, 1995a).

An example of the development+/planning mix is the National Institute for Women of Color. Its purpose, to "build a support network for and improve the self-esteem of women of color . . . to promote economic and educational well-being and to affirm the dignity of women of color" (Spalter-Roth & Schreiber, 1995, pp. 109, 116), clearly emphasizes development. It accomplishes its work through networking and self-help activities (development), and through the research and technical assistance attributed to social planning. Similarly, the Neighborhood Congress of Neighborhood Women offers training programs to enhance the skills of indigenous leaders (development) and to a relatively lesser extent investigates policies in terms of their affect on working class women (planning) (Reinharz, 1983).

Both the Project on Equal Rights (PEER), founded to monitor Title IX (sex equity law) enforcement, and the Displaced Homemakers Network, established to advocate for policies and programs favorable to displaced homemakers, illustrate the development/planning+ combination (Slater-Roth & Schreiber, 1995). While each offers some constituent training or education (e.g., how to monitor the implementation of the law), there is greater emphasis on data gathering, problem solving, and program planning to meet organizational goals. In their respective arenas, each organization acts as a type of citizen advisory board, the Rothman exemplar.

A feminist version of the planning/action combination is found in the Women's Equity Action League (WEAL). This organization lobbies in favor of feminist issues, monitors current sex-equity legislation enactment, and supports anti-discrimination litigation. Research and technical assistance provide the basis for such actions (Ferree & Hess, 1985). On a local level, the Connecticut Women's Educational and Legal Fund combines action in the form of organizing, information sharing, litigation, and lobbying with research to pursue its goal of sex equity in employment, education, and finance.

Rothman cites governmental planned reform as an expression of planning+/action. The state Commissions on the Status of Women are clear, feminist examples of this approach. These commissions, outgrowths of the President's [Kennedy] Commission on the Status of Women, were charged with "gathering data on the roles and resources of women and with documenting areas of discrimination in the laws and practices of individual states" (Ferree & Hess, 1985, p. 53). Through these processes, however, a more latent goal of action, specifically education, public hearings, and legislative efforts, emerged. Similarly, the Radcliffe Public Policy Institute seeks to change public policy through research on women's lives. These research efforts, however, have a decidedly action orientation ("Statement of purpose: Radcliffe . . . ", n.d.).

Finally, the planning/action+ example of the Women's Action Coalition suggests the radical possibilities of this combination. Through public demonstrations and media campaigns, this organization fulfills its mission of "an open alliance of women committed to DIRECT ACTION on issues affecting the rights of all women. . . . We will exercise our full creative power to launch a visible and remarkable resistance" (WAC, 1993, p. 2). This organization also publishes a compilation of research findings, called *WAC Stats,* in order to systematically illustrate the plight of women globally. Though not as far reaching in scope, the Italian League for Divorce successfully fought for liberal divorce laws in Italy by "using political pressure tactics that have become the trademark of the Italian Radical Party" (Beckwith, 1987, p. 157). This mobilization effort, however, was grounded in careful research that suggested both the need for and possibility of reform, and it was conducted within a policy arena.

This revision of Rothman's Figure 1.5 ought to suggest the organizational scope of feminism in the last 30 years. The movement's breadth, specifically the variations in approaches all under the banner of feminism, is clear. Thus, this effort represents a corrective to Rothman's designation of feminist enterprises. And, it should further clarify just what Rothman means when he speaks of the various models and their combinations. Yet beyond these descriptive functions, what is learned from this effort?

IMPLICATIONS FOR COMMUNITY PRACTICE ANALYSIS

This discussion of feminist approaches to community intervention raises several questions and concerns for the broader field of macro practice analysis. While perhaps inspiring in its own right, designating feminist versions of Rothman's examples is not just an exercise in mentioning as many interesting organizations as possible. It also is not an admonishment that more feminist examples should have been included; indeed, the range of organizations mentioned by Rothman ought to be appreciated. The larger purpose of this effort was to lift up for discussion some concerns with Rothman's (and others') approach to community intervention, in particular, and with the state of macro practice scholarship, in general.

In doing this revision exercise, the author was surprised by how difficult it was to place most of the organizations. Many of the feminist projects exhibited all three intervention modes, suggesting more overlap and indeterminateness than conveyed by Rothman. Rothman's primary interest is the creation and comparison of intervention types, yet several important assumptions, as well as ambiguities, that undergird his categorizations go unacknowledged. These were revealed by virtue of engaging in the revision process.

First, there is scant attention in Rothman's account to the role of ideology within intervention types. It is well into the paper before he notes that the inclusion of an ideological dimension to the social action model would be a worthwhile revision to the discussion of goals. Yet he limits its import by noting that this addition is "tactical in nature" (this volume, p. 93) and by considering it only for the action model and not the other two. Ideology, however, is crucial in terms of shaping the visions of the interventions and of attendant organizations. Ideologies convey basic values and beliefs, provide rationales for membership, promote cohesion, and guide strategies–the philosophical glue, if you will. An organization's ideology shapes the development of goals, structures, processes and outcomes (Hyde, 1992; 1995a/b). Within feminism, ideological disputes (and at times battles) have long existed–liberal vs. radical vs. socialist vs. cultural. These different ideological perspectives often result in different strategies (e.g., working in coalitions) and organizational types (e.g., bureaucratic or collective) (Hyde, 1992). Other movements no doubt wage similar debates, though one would not know this from much of the community intervention literature which is distinctly non-ideological.

Rothman implicitly entertains ideology in his references to revolutionary strategy under the auspices of social action. Yet in this regard, he equates revolution with the stereotypically militant, "take to the street" techniques, conceiving it as only an aspect of action interventions. Feminism approaches revolution, or revolutionary potential, differently. Feminist theorist Charlotte Bunch (1974) argues that we should move away from style distinctions (lobbying vs. bombing) and instead examine substantive content and ultimate goals. In this sense, revolution is about "a total restructuring of the ideology and institutions of the society" (p. 39) and may be pursued through various strategies, including reforms, so long as they advance and expand the power of the constituent group (e.g., women). Moreover, feminists understand revolution as a long, evolutionary process involving continuous challenges to the status quo. Thus, feminist organizations that deliver services, such as a health clinic, are revolutionary in that they confront fundamental assumptions regarding the delivery of care (Hyde, 1992). Despite this revolutionary stance, these organizations do not fit Rothman's action mode, because of the way in which he has limited the meaning of revolution.

Also tied to ideology are the dimensions of process and task. Rothman dichotomizes these properties, noting that social planning embraces task goals; locality development, process goals; and social action, both task and process. In reality, intervention modes, as cultivated in organizations, pursue both types of goals. And, these goals are shaped by the overarching ideological frame. Process, or reflexive, goals focus on such internal, maintenance activities as governance, decision making, and personnel development. Task, or transitive, goals target organizational activities in the environment, such as tangible products and services (Hyde, 1992). Therefore, feminist (and other) organizations cannot be categorized in this way. What can be learned from feminist endeavors is how these two goals are balanced, when emphasis on one over another ought to occur, and what happens when one inappropriately dominates the other (e.g., co-optation).

What made the categorization of the feminist organizational examples so difficult was that these dimensions (ideology, revolutionary orientation, process and task) vary depending on the age of the organization. That is, newer organizations may orient towards one style of intervention, while veteran organizations will settle into another mode. While Rothman mentions that a mixing and phasing of approaches occurs (this volume, p. 94), he greatly underestimates the importance of such processes. The vast majority of the feminist examples embraced different modes, usually over time, but sometimes simultaneously. Rothman's desire for categorization, a desire well shared in the field, relies on "freezing" the organization in time. But what of the lessons of longitudinal analysis–when and why do certain modality mixes or phasings occur, what are the patterns, and what are the consequences? Such questions are obscured by categorization schemes; this is unfortunate given the rich literature on organizational developmental stages that could have been used (Child & Kieser, 1981; Feree & Martin, 1995b; Hyde, 1992; Morris & Mueller, 1992; Staggenborg, 1989; Whetton, 1987; Zald & McCarthy, 1987; Zald & Ash, 1973).

Fundamentally, there is a lack of clarity regarding the unit of analysis. What does Rothman, indeed what do other community practice scholars, mean to examine when the focus is on "community intervention"? Rothman's unit of analysis often is not community intervention; at least, not community intervention as a process. Rather, his focus is on organizations that embrace intervention goals. This accounts for the initial confusion between feminist organizing and illustrative organizational expressions of intervention types. This confusion remains throughout much of Rothman's presentation; it is often not clear whether he is speaking of organizational properties or larger movement ones. He is not alone; the field is replete with examples that confound mobilization processes with organizational types.

Also not clear in Rothman's discussion is what is meant by community. Rothman seems to mean all or part of a geographic community (see Table 1, this volume, pp. 72-73), yet his organizational illustrations suggest otherwise. Rubin and Rubin suggest several types of community, based on type of integration promoted, including: the neighborhood with geographic boundaries; the solidarity community with a common heritage or background; the social class community based on economic or work status; the social network premised on shared interests; and the community of interest from solidarity through collective action (1986, p. 37). By virtue of his examples, Rothman moves between neighborhood and interest forms of community. This lacks clarity, however, and one wonders whether types of communities and intervention modalities combine in particular ways. Here again, feminist analysis provides some insights, as certain ideological perspectives shape the understanding of community (e.g., liberal feminist–social network community; socialist feminist–combined class and interest community) (Hyde, 1995a).

In all these areas of concern, the community practice field's failure to tap the sociology of social movement literature is particularly telling. Exceptions aside (e.g., Fisher, 1994; Fisher & Kling, 1994; Hyde, 1992, 1995a/b), community intervention scholars make little use of social movement analysis and instead, focus more on case descriptions and typologies. If organizations are the focus, then the extensive studies on social movement organizations would illuminate, in a more complex and analytical way, the pivotal role that (usually indigenous) organizations play in mobilization efforts (for example, see Ferree & Martin, 1995a, 1995b; Zald & McCarthy, 1987). Clarity would be gained as to how various organizations properties–ideology, goals, structures and processes, products, external relations–differentially shape outcomes over time. If horizons are broadened to incorporate more on larger movement dynamics, insights from the social movement literature on identity politics, advances and backlash, co-optation, protest cycles, coalitions and infrastructure (for example, see Melucci, 1989; Morris & Mueller, 1992) would be garnered. Neglecting the social movement literature greatly diminishes an understanding of the what's, why's, and how's of community practice.

Despite these concerns, Rothman has mounted a comprehensive and detailed effort. Yet, there remains one lingering problem with his overall approach. Despite, or perhaps because of, his expansive presentation, the core of community intervention is lost. That core is one of passionate and vibrant commitment (Hirsch, 1990; Hyde, 1994). The absence of this characteristic was acutely felt when the list of feminist examples was compiled. There seemed to be no room for this realm, so central to feminist endeavors. Yet heart-felt commitment does not belong exclusively to feminism. Rather, through the analysis presented in this paper, its absence is underscored; the extension of this analysis suggests that with the tendency to categorize community interventions, the dynamism of commitment is lost. Yet that is the very reason why so many engage in this work. Without the inclusion of passion in this, or any other, analysis, community practitioners have only a partial understanding of their world.

NOTES

1. Rothman (1995) notes that the article first appeared in 1968. This author became acquainted with his 1979 version at the beginning of her MSW program in 1981.

2. When discussing intervention combinations, such as action/development, the "+" indicates which of the two modes is dominant.

REFERENCES

Beckwith, K. (1987). Response to feminism in the Italian parliament: Divorce, abortion, and sexual violence legislation. In M. Katzenstein & C. Mueller (Eds.), *The women's movements of the United States and Western Europe*, (pp. 153-171). Philadelphia: Temple University Press.

Brandwein, R. (1981). Toward the feminization of community and organization practice. *Social Development Issues*, *5*, 180-193.

Brilliant, E. (1990). *The United Way: Dilemmas of organized charity*. New York: Columbia University Press.

Buehler, J. (1985). The Puget Sound women's peace camp: Education as an alternative strategy. *Frontiers*, *VII*(2), 40-44.

Bunch, C. (1974). The reform tool kit. *Quest I*(1), 37-64.

Child, J., & Kieser, A. (1981). Development of organizations over time. In P. Nystrom and W. Starbuck (Eds.), *Handbook of organizational design*, vol. 1 (pp. 28-64). New York: Oxford University Press.

de Bretteville, S. (1980). The Los Angeles woman's building: A public center for woman's culture. In G. Werlele (Ed.), *New space for women* (pp. 293-310). Boulder: Westview Press.

Eisenstein, H. (1995). The Australian femocratic experiment: A feminist case for bureaucracy. In M. M. Ferree & P. Martin (Eds.), *Feminist organizations: Harvest of the new women's movement* (pp. 69-83). Philadelphia: Temple University Press.

Elam, P. (1989). The militant state of mind: Organizing the Congressional Union, Inc. *Women's Studies International Forum*, *12*(1), 101-105.

Ferree, M. & Hess, B. (1985). *Controversy and coalition: The new feminist movement*. Boston: Twayne Publishers.

Ferree, M. & Martin, P. (1995a). Doing the work of the movement: Feminist organizations. In M. M. Ferree & P. Martin (Eds.), *Feminist organizations: Harvest of the new women's movement* (pp. 3-26). Philadelphia: Temple University Press.

Ferree, M., & Martin, P. (Eds.) (1995b). *Feminist organizations: Harvest of the new women's movement*. Philadelphia: Temple University Press.

Fisher, R. (1994). *Let the people decide*. Boston: Twayne.

Fisher, R., & Kling, J. (1994). Community organization and new social movements theory. *Journal of Progressive Human Service*, *59*(2), 5-24.

Garland, A. W. (1988). *Women activists: Challenging the abuse of power*. New York: The Feminist Press.

Gutierrez, L. M. & Lewis, E. (1992). A feminist perspective on organizing with women of color. In F. Rivera & J. Erlich (Eds.), *Community organizing in a diverse society* (pp. 113-132). Needham Heights, MA: Allyn & Bacon.

Hirsch, E. L. (1990). Sacrifice for the cause: Group processes, recruitment, and commitment in a student social movement. *American Sociological Review*, *55*, 243-262.

Hyde, C. (1995a). Feminist social movement organizations survive the New Right. In M. M. Ferree & P. Martin (Eds.), *Feminist organizations: Harvest of the new women's movement* (pp. 306-322). Philadelphia: Temple University Press.

Hyde, C. (1995b). The politics of authority. In N. Van Den Bergh (Ed.), *Feminist social work for the 21st century* (pp. 89-102). Washington, DC: NASW Press.

Hyde, C. (1994). Commitment to social change: Voices from the feminist movement. *Journal of Community Practice*, *1*(2), 45-64.

Hyde, C. (1992). The ideational system of social movement agencies: An examination of feminist health centers. In Y. Hasenfeld (Ed.), *Human services as complex organizations* (pp. 121-144). Newbury Park: Sage Publications.

Hyde, C. (1989). A feminist model for macro-practice: Promises and problems. *Administration in Social Work, 13*, 145-181.

I cry for help, No one's there . . . (n.d.). Brochure. Bangalore, India: Vimochana.

Martin, P. (1990). Rethinking feminist organizations. *Gender & Society, 4*, 182-206.

Melucci, A. (1989). *Nomads of the present: Social movements and individual needs in contemporary society.* Philadelphia: Temple University Press.

Morris, A., & Mueller, C. (Eds.) (1992). *Frontiers in social movement theory.* New Haven: Yale University Press.

Reinharz, S. (1983). Women as competent community builders. *Issues in Mental Health Nursing 5*, 19-43.

Rothman, J. (1996). The Interweaving of Community Intervention Approaches. *Journal of Community Practice, 3(3/4)*, 69-99.

Rothman, J. (1995). Approaches to community intervention. In J. Rothman, J. Erlich, J. Tropman & F. Cox (Eds.), *Strategies of community intervention* (pp. 26-63). Itasca, IL: Peacock Publishers.

Rothman, J. (1979). Three models of community organization practice, their mixing and phasing. In F. Cox, J. Erlich, J. Rothman, & J. Tropman (Eds.), *Strategies of community organizing* (pp. 25-44). Itasca, IL: Peacock Publishers.

Rubin, H. & Rubin, I. (1986). *Community organizing and development.* Columbus, OH: Merrill Publishing.

Sargent, M. (1989). Women rising in resistance: A direct action network. *Women's Studies International Forum, 12*(1), 113-118.

Searles, P. & Berger, R. J. (1987). The feminist self-defense movement: A case study. *Gender & Society, 1*(1), 61-84.

Slater-Roth, R. & Schreiber, R. (1995). Outsider issues and insider tactics: Strategic tensions in the women's policy network during the 1980s. In M. M. Ferree & P. Martin (Eds.), *Feminist organizations: Harvest of the new women's movement* (pp. 105-127). Philadelphia: Temple University Press.

Staggenborg, S. (1989). Stability and innovation in the women's movement: A comparison of two movement organizations. *Social Problems, 36*(1), 75-92.

Statement of purpose: Chicago Women's Liberation Union (n.d.). Chicago: Chicago Women's Liberation Union.

Statement of purpose: Radcliffe Policy Institute (n.d.). Cambridge: Radcliffe Public Policy Institute, Radcliffe College.

Strobel, M. (1995). Organizational learning in the Chicago women's liberation union. In M. M. Ferree & P. Martin (Eds.), *Feminist organizations: Harvest of the new women's movement* (pp. 145-164). Philadelphia: Temple University Press.

Weil, M. (1988). Creating an alternative work culture in a public service setting. *Administration in Social Work, 12*(2), 69-82.

Weil, M. (1986). Women, community, and organizing. In N. Van Den Bergh & L. Cooper (Eds.), *Feminist visions for social work* (pp. 187-210). Silver Springs: NASW Press.

Whetton, D. A. (1987). Organizational growth and decline processes. *Annual Review of Sociology, 13*, 335-358.
Women's Action Coalition (1993). *WAC stats: The facts about women*. New York: The New Press.
Zald, M. & McCarthy, J. (Eds.) (1987). *Social movements in an organizational society.* New Brunswick, NJ: Transaction Books.
Zald, M. & Ash, R. (1973). Social movement organizations: Growth, decay, and change. In R. Evans (Eds.), *Social movements: A reader and source book* (pp. 80-102). Chicago: Rand McNally.

Community Work: British Models

Keith Popple, PhD

SUMMARY. This article presents a typology of models of community work currently extant in the United Kingdom. It focuses on clarifying theoretical points through analysis of the currently most widely accepted contemporary models in use throughout the UK: community care; community organization; community development; social/community planning; community education; and community action, and developing models of feminist community work, and black and anti-racist community work. The typology presented is organized on a continuum from models focused on "care" to those focusing on "action." Each model is analyzed in relation to the following characteristics: strategy; workers' main roles; and typical agencies and examples of work. Selected critical key texts treating each model are documented. Discussion highlights similarities and differences among the models particularly with regard to techniques and skills and ideological traditions to provide a framework to understand community work practice.

Keith Popple is Senior Lecturer in Social Policy in the Department of Social Policy and Social Work, University of Plymouth, United Kingdom.

Address correspondence to: Keith Popple, Department of Social Policy and Social Work, University of Plymouth, Drake Circus, Plymouth, Devon PL4 8AA, United Kingdom.

This article was originally published as a chapter entitled "Models of Community Work" in *Analysing Community Work: Its Theory and Practice* (1995), Buckingham: Open University Press. Reprinted with permission. *Analysing Community Work* is available from Taylor & Francis Inc. in the U.S., price US $24.95 pb and US $79.00 cloth.

[Haworth co-indexing entry note]: "Community Work: British Models." Popple, Keith. Co-published simultaneously in *Journal of Community Practice* (The Haworth Press, Inc.) Vol. 3, No. 3/4, 1996, pp. 147-180; and: *Community Practice: Conceptual Models* (ed: Marie Weil) The Haworth Press, Inc., 1996, pp. 147-180.

KEYWORDS. Community practice models, United Kingdom community practice, community work

Community work comprises both theory and practice, and although they are inextricably linked, for our own purposes it is more productive initially to consider each of them separately. The focus of this article is to reflect upon the theoretical understandings already developed by analysing the models which constitute contemporary community work practice. This in turn helps to distinguish community work from other forms of intervention.

An extensive review of the community work literature fails to provide an agreed number or the exact scope of different community work models. What has been developed here, therefore, is a discussion that includes the models most readily agreed upon: community care, community organization, community development, social/community planning, community education and community action, together with models developed from feminist community work theory and the black and anti-racist critique. It will be noted that these models have evolved often in an uncoordinated manner to address a particular difficulty or concern, or as the application of a particular theory or approach. It needs to be recognized that aspects of these models are not entirely discrete, but rather there is a degree of overlap between them. The models are, however, an important method of categorizing central approaches to the activity we call "community work." They have been ordered on a continuum from those concerned primarily with "care" to those known for their emphasis on "action." This provides a helpful way of contrasting and comparing the models. Table 1 provides a typology.

COMMUNITY CARE

Community work which is focused on the model of community care attempts to cultivate social networks and voluntary services for, or to be concerned about, the welfare of residents, particularly older people, persons with disabilities, and in many cases children under the age of five. The community care model concentrates on developing self-help concepts to address social and welfare needs

TABLE 1. Models of community work practice.

	Strategy	*Main role/title of worker*	*Examples of work/ agencies*	*Selected critical key texts*
Community Care	Cultivating social networks and voluntary services Developing self-help concepts	Organizer Volunteer	Work with older people, persons with disabilities, children under 5 years	Beresford and Croft (1986)
Community organization	Improving co-ordination between different welfare agencies	Organizer Catalyst Manager	Councils for Voluntary Service Racial Equality Councils Settlements	Adamson et al. (1988) Dearlove (1974) Dominelli (1990)
Community development	Assisting groups to acquire the skills and confidence to improve quality of life Active participation	Enabler Neighbourhood worker Facilitator	Community groups Tenants groups Settlements	Association of Metropolitan Authorities (1993) Barr (1991)
Social/ community planning	Analysis of social conditions, setting of goals and priorities, implementing and evaluating services and programmes	Enabler Facilitator	Localities undergoing redevelopment	Marris (1987) Twelvetrees (1991)
Community education	Attempts to bring education and community into a closer and more equal relationship	Educator Facilitator	Community schools/colleges 'Compensatory education' Working-class/feminist adult education	Allen et al. (1987) Allen and Martin (1992) Freire (1970; 1972; 1976; 1985) Lovett (1975) Lovett et al. (1983) Rogers (1994)
Community action	Usually class-based, conflict-focused direct action at local level	Activist	Squatting movement Welfare rights movement Resistance against planning and redevelopment Tenants' action	CDP literature (see Appendix A) Craig et al. (1982) Jacobs and Popple (1994) Lees and Mayo (1984)

TABLE 1 (continued)

	Strategy	*Main role/title of worker*	*Examples of work/ agencies*	*Selected critical key texts*
Feminist community work	Improvement of women's welfare Working collectively to challenge and eradicate inequalities suffered by women	Activist Enabler Facilitator	Women's refuges Women's health groups Women's therapy centres	Barker (1986) Dixon et al. (1982) Dominelli (1990; 1994) Flynn et al. (1986)
Black and anti-racist community work	Setting up and running groups that support the needs of black people. Challenging racism	Activist Volunteer	Racial Equality Councils and Commission for Racial Equality funded projects	Ohri et al. (1982) Sivanandan (1976; 1990) Sondhi (1982; 1994)

and uses paid workers (sometimes termed 'organizers') who encourage people to care and to volunteer initiative. Professional involvement in community care can be on one of three levels. One level is where professionals are expected to fulfil a more or less permanent supportive or monitoring role, using volunteers and low-paid helpers. A second level is where the activity is initiated by professionals who plan to be supportive for only a short period, so that community care can be continued without them. A third level reflects community care as an activity undertaken by laypeople with relatively little help from professionals.

The voluntarism associated with the community care model supports the notion of engaging volunteers in care-giving (and advocacy schemes). In reality, there may be concerns over the level of training of volunteers and their reliability. Similarly, there may be concern about the exploitation of volunteers as free labour, which may also serve to undermine the jobs of paid workers.

In practice, the term 'informal care' refers to care undertaken by families, neighbours and friends, on an informal, unpaid basis and largely in the recipients' own homes. The important contribution of this sector has been recognised for some time. It has been estimated that the value of informal care ranges from ***L*** 15 to ***L*** 24 billion per year (Family Policy Studies Centre, 1989). Such calculations are very difficult to make with any accuracy as the defining feature of this sector is its informal and largely hidden nature. The figures were, however, arrived at using a notional rate of ***L*** 4 per hour, irrespective of the level of care provided. This calculation takes no account of the additional expenditures (travel, adaptations, etc.) or of the opportunity costs in terms of careers and wages foregone by carers. Neither does it take any account of costs of childcare. The figure is useful, however, if only to offer an illustration of this sector's contribution in comparison to total government expenditure on social services in 1987-8 amounting to ***L*** 3.34 billion (HM Treasury, 1987).

An optimistic view of the role of volunteers in community care is provided by Heginbotham (1990), who argues that a 'communitarian' approach to community care empowers people through their defining and participating in services for their own needs. He argues for a new vision of volunteering in which local services are managed by local people, an argument also persuasively made by Beresford and Croft (1986). Cutting across the arguments posited by different political groupings, Heginbotham (1990: 42) believes that there needs to be a balance between

> individual worth with collective responsibility, to fuse liberal economic ideals with market socialism, and to recognise the interplay between the central and local state, on the one hand, and the community (often represented by voluntary organizations) on the other.

Heginbotham's laudable brave new world will attract few dissenters although his thesis has few practical examples of how it would work, and does not convincingly counter the criticism that a central tenet of the drive in the 1980s and 1990s towards community care can be viewed as minimizing state welfare expenditure (Walker, 1989).

Numerous studies have supported the view that women are much more likely to be engaged in community care than men (Croft, 1986; Equal Opportunities Commission, 1984; Finch and Groves, 1983; Lewis and Meredith, 1990; Ungerson, 1987). These findings are also reported by Parker (1981, 31) who states that to talk about community or family care is to 'disguise reality':

> In fact, . . . 'care by the community' almost always means care by family members with little support from others in the 'com-

> munity'. Further care by family members almost always means care by female members with little support from other relatives. It appears that 'shared care' is uncommon; once one person has been identified as the main carer other relatives withdraw.

Community care policies have been criticised by a number of social policy writers who point to the dominance of familist ideology, and its links with the wider ideology of possessive individualism (Dalley, 1988; Finch, 1984; Finch and Groves, 1985; Wicks, 1987). Dalley, for instance, argues that community care has been actively promoted by the Right for a number of reasons. These usually revolve around the need to avoid the expense of institutional care, but also because this form of care is perceived as the most 'appropriate' and 'natural' form of care for the dependent. This view is derived from the residualist or anti-collectivist approach to welfare whereby the family is seen as the locus of care, and the role of the statutory sector only comes into play when that unit has broken down in some way. The Barclay (1982), Griffiths (1988) and Wagner (1988) reports developed the policy and practice of community care models, endorsing the early development of localizing social work services that had been taking place in some areas (Hadley and Hatch, 1981; Hadley and McGrath, 1980), while hastening the development of community-based social work in local authorities elsewhere. The intention throughout was for social work departments to account more effectively for, and deliver, their services in the changing political, social and economic climate (Hadley et al., 1987).

Considerable discussion has been allocated here to the community care model. This is because during the late 1980s and the 1990s the model rapidly developed as a significant and relatively well-resourced form of community work which had clear connections with the ascendancy and influence of the New Right ideology of the same period (Leavitas, 1986; Loney et al., 1991). However, it needs to be noted that since the 1960s a number of social scientists have developed a critique of the failure of institutional care to provide people with humane treatment (Foucault, 1967, 1977; Goffman, 1961; Jones and Fowles, 1984; Morris, 1969; Robb, 1967; Scull,

1977; Townsend, 1962), while more recently the UK disability movement has stressed the desire of disabled people for independent living in mainstream housing rather than institutional care (Morris, 1990).

COMMUNITY ORGANIZATION

Community work formulated on the community organization model has been used widely in Britain as a means of improving the co-ordination between different welfare agencies. Through such co-ordination it is thought possible to avoid duplication of services and poverty of resources while attempting to provide an efficient and effective delivery of welfare. Examples of community organizations are councils of voluntary service, older person's welfare committees, and 'similar organizations that are engaged in the co-ordination, promotion and development of the work of a number of bodies in a particular field at local, regional or national levels' (Jones, 1977: 6). The community organization model, which tends to be service-oriented, has been engaged in pioneering and experimental work and has often led to the state funding and managing the services developed by such organizations (Kramer, 1979).

Most critics of the community organization model underpin their arguments with theories from the radical and socialist approach. They include Dearlove (1974), who has cited the role of community organizations in employing 'expert' professionals whose job it is to offer advice to working-class people in an attempt to stifle the anger and frustration felt in a particular locality or community. The role of the 'expert' in this model is to channel these feelings into acceptable and approved structures. Dominelli (1990) takes up this point, arguing that community organization has been used by the local state in rationing its declining resource base. The Community Development Projects were also critical of the community organization mode. They argued, for instance, that the Urban Deprivation Unit created by the Department of Environment in 1973 was based on the community organization model, operating with managerialist methods, and ignoring the needs and concerns of people living in the communities they professed to serve (CDP, 1977). Feminists have similarly criticized the community organization model (Dominelli, 1990: 10), although there has been evidence of feminists developing new styles of community organization (Adamson et al., 1988).

COMMUNITY DEVELOPMENT

The community development model of community work is concerned with assisting groups to acquire the skills and confidence to improve the quality of the lives of its members. With its emphasis on promoting self-help by means of education, this model is thought to reflect the 'uniqueness of community work' (Twelvetrees, 1991: 98). The community development model, which was championed in North America in the early 1960s by Biddle and Biddle (1965), evolved in Britain from the work initiated by Batten (1957, 1962, 1965, 1967) which initially derived from his experiences with such a model when working in the colonies. This model of community work was used as a tool by British administrations overseas to harness the local communities into colonial domination. The rationale for the model being used by the British Colonial Office can be seen in HMSO (1954), while a similar notion is given in the United Nations statement on community development in developing countries (United Nations, 1959: 1). The use of the community development model in developing countries has been criticised by Ng (1988), who documents how the model was used in the colonies to integrate black people into subordinate positions within the dominant colonizing system.

The experience of community development in Britain has been characterized by work at the neighbourhood level and, as noted earlier, has focused upon a process whereby community groups are encouraged to articulate their problems and needs. The expectation is that this will lead to collective action in the determination and meeting of these needs. The typical worker in this model has been described by Dominelli (1990: 11) as 'usually a man who helps people learn by working on problems they have identified. He is typically a paid professional interested in reforming the system through social engineering.'

There are, of course, numerous examples of women being employed as community development workers. For example, a black woman, Anionwu (1990), has written up her community development work in relation to a marginalized health problem, sickle cell anaemia. Anionwu believes that the community development approach was successful in enabling her to meet and work with discriminated black sufferers, which led to her setting up the Brent Sickle Cell and Thalassic Centre.

Barr (1991) reviews and analyses Strathclyde Regional Council's programme of community development which is considered to be the most substantial of its kind in British local government. Discussion of his two field studies of the Social Work Department's community workers leads Barr to consider the role and practice of community development as a major policy initiative. In his findings Barr (1991: 166) argues that community development has a legitimate part to play in providing opportunities for 'radical alliances of professional, political and community interests to promote redistributive, anti-deprivation policies and practices.' Similarly, Roberts (1992) argues that community development workers based in local authority social services departments are in a position to contribute to the establishment and practice of imaginative community care proposals. He believes the skills and knowledge that are inherent in the community development model can be used to provide opportunities for people to achieve power and control over their own lives. This, he argues, will give community development a role within local government administration where the practice is under threat.

In his own work Barr draws the conclusion that community development workers would be more effective if they laid more emphasis upon social planning approaches. This was a concept established by Rothman (1976), who placed community development alongside social planning, and this has since been developed by Twelvetrees (1991). Twelvetrees (1991: 7) argues that whereas community development is involved in working alongside a particular community (whether locality or community of interest), social planning involves the community worker 'liaising and working directly with policy-makers and service providers to improve services or alter policies.' In some typologies of community work, and in particular those developed by Jones (1977), Rothman (1976), Thomas (1983) and Twelvetrees (1991), social planning is considered to be a discrete model of community work and it is to this area we now turn.

Social/Community Planning

As noted above, the social/community planning model of community work is considered to be similar to community development and has been described as

> the analysis of social conditions, social policies and agency services; the setting of goals and priorities; the design of service programmes and the mobilisation of appropriate resources; and the implementation and evaluation of services and programmes. (Thomas, 1983: 109)

The social/community planning model is believed to be the most common of community work models (Twelvetrees, 1991: 98). However, as Twelvetrees points out, this is complicated by the breadth of the term 'social/community planning,' which can include economic planning and national planning. According to Twelvetrees, this means that although most community workers are engaged in social/community planning, not all those involved in this activity can be termed 'community workers.'

One of the advocates of social/community planning, which he calls simply 'community planning,' is Marris (1987), who argues that it should be possible to incorporate the demand for open, democratic planning into political struggles for social justice. Marris believes that the failure of the Community Development Projects was due in part to their classical Marxist analysis of class relations which failed to recognize the subtle, complex and changing nature of working-class communities. He also believes that this focus on class antagonism led to an inability to work within the state to achieve improvements for the people who lived in the neighbourhoods the projects were intended to assist. Instead, Marris argues that if community work is to effect anything more than marginal change it needs to find common ground with the government even if the ideologies of the two are at variance. Marris suggests that social/community planning is one strategy that can be used to help protect working-class communities from the uncertainty and lack of control they suffer when redevelopment takes place in their locality. In Marris's view, then, community workers, including radical community workers, have more to gain for the communities they serve by developing a partnership with the state, and by practising the community planning model.

The main criticism that can be levelled at this view is that it assumes that the knowledge gained by community workers will be used by decision-makers in a rational manner for the benefit of the members of the community in question. Evidence from Marris is not entirely convincing. For example, he cites the redevelopment of London's docklands and the evolution of the Docklands Strategic Plan which attempted to involve and take account of the people living in the affected area (Newham Docklands Forum and Greater London Council Popular Planning Unit, 1983). He later admits, however, that the plan actually had little effect because

> plans are so often ignored, whenever they attempt to set priorities and guarantees in the interests of the most vulnerable, or constrain the freedom of action of those more powerful so as to reach some resolution which is both fair and practicable [so that], planning even at its best often comes to seem merely a distraction from more effective forms of political protest, and so co-optive. (Marris, 1987, 160)

However, Marris continues to believe in the potential of the social/community planning model because political struggle without it leads only to 'competitive bargaining between different kinds of interests, and that cannot protect the weaker and more vulnerable members of society' (Marris, 1987: 160).

Community Education

The community education model of community work has been described as 'a significant attempt to redirect educational policy and practice in ways which bring education and community into a closer and more equal relationship' (Allen et al., 1987: 2). Community education has a long tradition in the United Kingdom which, according to I. Martin (1987), has evolved from three main strands. The first is the school-based village and community college movement initiated by Henry Morris in Cambridgeshire during the late 1920s (Morris, 1925). (For discussion on the life and work of Morris see Ree, 1973, 1985.) This was followed by the establishment of similar integrated educational provision in Leicestershire under the guidance of Stewart Mason during the following decade (Fairbairn, 1979). The second strand of community education were the experiments developing from the Educational Priority Area projects (1969-72) which attempted to provide 'compensatory education' in selected disadvantaged inner-city areas as recommended by DES (1967). (For a detailed discussion of these experiments, see also Halsey, 1972; Midwinter, 1972, 1975.) The third strand was the working-class adult education work undertaken by a number of the Community Development Projects in the late 1960s and the early 1970s (for example, see Lovett, 1975; Lovett et al., 1983).

Community education has been further analysed as having three 'qualitatively different ideologies': consensus, pluralism, and conflict (I. Martin, 1987: 22). Martin argues that the consensus or universal model is focused around the secondary school/community college; the pluralist or reformist model is linked to primary schools and their neighbourhoods; and the conflict or radical model is focused around working-class action. To this can be added the feminist analysis of community education which is clearly articulated by Rogers (1994). The conflict or radical model shares with community development an emphasis on innovative, informal, political education, and has been greatly influenced by the Brazilian adult educator, Paulo Freire, whose work has served as a significant challenge to school-based education. It is because of his influence upon the practice of community work that we need to consider Freire's work in greater detail.

Working with poverty-stricken South American communities during the 1960s, Freire, who at the present time is resident professor of education at the University of Sao Paulo, Brazil, and visiting professor at Havard's Centre for Studies in Education and Development, found ways of developing approaches by which people can express their feelings and experiences. He developed an educational process which rejects the traditional hierarchical 'banking system,' where knowledge is considered to be a commodity accumulated in order to gain access to positions of power and privilege. In its place

Freire developed an 'education for liberation' where learners and teachers engage in a process in which abstract and concrete knowledge, together with experience, are integrated into *praxis* (which can be defined as action intended to alter the material and social world). The fundamental features of this praxis are critical thinking and dialogue (as opposed to discussion) which seek to challenge conventional explanations of everyday life, while at the same time considering the action necessary for the transformation of oppressive conditions.

The extensive work of Freire (1970, 1972, 1976, 1985) centres on the concept of 'conscientization,' otherwise known as politicization and political action. According to Freire, before people can engage in action for change they have first to reflect upon their present situation. However, the nature of ideological domination means that subordinate groups accept, and frequently collude with, the reproduction of a society's inequalities and explanations and justifications offered for the status, power and privilege of their oppressors: an idea similar to notions developed by Gramsci. Overcoming this false ideology means overcoming people's pessimistic and fatalistic thinking. Freire understood this was not an easy task, but his great optimism and purpose have led to educators around the world taking up the challenge.

Freire believes that educators have to work on the wide range of experiences brought by oppressed people. The educational process entails providing opportunities for people to validate their experiences, culture, dreams, values and histories, while recognizing that such expressions carry both the seeds of radical change and the burden of oppression. Freire's position coincides with that held by many community workers that it is necessary to start from a person's own understanding. According to Freire, the skill is to work with people by a 'problematizing' approach rather than a 'problem-solving' stance as advocated in the banking system of education. 'Problem-solving' involves an expert being distant from a person's reality while engaging in an analysis that efficiently resolves difficulties before dictating a strategy of policy. Freire believes that this reduces human experience and difficulties to that which can be 'treated.' 'Problematizing,' however, means immersing oneself in the struggle of disadvantaged communities and engaging in the task 'of codifying total reality into symbols which can generate critical consciousness' (Freire, 1976: ix).

According to Freire, this empowers people to begin to alter their social relations. Freire believes that this is undertaken by a process of critical reflection and action followed by further critical reflection and action. This, he continues, creates conditions for the development of genuine theory and collective action because both are rooted in historical and cultural reality. However, Freire believes that theory and practice are not conflated into one another. Instead, there needs to be a distance between the two. 'Theory does not dictate practice; rather, it serves to hold practice at arm's length in order to mediate and critically comprehend the type of praxis needed within a specific setting at a particular time in history' (Freire, 1985: xxiii).

Allman (1987) believes that Freire's ideas have begun to permeate liberal education in the United Kingdom but because of the structure and underlying ideology of the present system they are likely to be used only selectively. Similarly, Allman (1987: 214) argues that Freire's ideas have been distorted and devalued in the 'futile attempt to incorporate "radical" technique in the "liberal" agenda.' Taking note of these criticisms, Freire's work, together with the writings of Gramsci, has implications for the theory and practice of community work.

COMMUNITY ACTION

The community action model of community work is both a reaction to the more paternalistic forms of community work and a response by relatively powerless groups to increase their effectiveness. In Britain, the Community Development Projects were initiated as a government-supported community work venture based upon the community organization and community development models. Soon after their commencement this direction changed, with the Projects evolving on the lines of the community action model.

The community action model of community work has traditionally been class-based and uses conflict and direct action, usually at a local level, in order to negotiate with power holders over what is often a single issue. Early writings on community action by, among others, Lapping (1970), Leonard (1975), Radford (1970), and Silburn (1971), together with the influential community work series of books published by Routledge and Kegan Paul in conjunction with the Association of Community Workers (Craig et al., 1979, 1982; Curno, 1978; Jones and Mayo, 1975; Mayo, 1977; Mayo and Jones, 1974; Ohri et al., 1982; Smith and Jones, 1981), as well as a number of other significant writings (for example Cockburn, 1977; Cowley et al., 1977; Curno et al., 1982; Lees and Mayo, 1984; O'Malley, 1977) provide a rich source of examples of the practice and debates surrounding the model during the late 1960s, 1970s and early 1980s. The North American community work literature also contains examples and discussions of community or social action. The texts that have been the most influential in the United Kingdom include Alinsky (1969, 1971), Lamoureux et al. (1989), and Piven and Cloward (1977).

Since the 1960s examples of community action have been varied and include the squatting movement, the welfare rights movement (including the Claimants Union), and different forms of resistance against planning and redevelopment. Mayo (1982) believes the most typical form of community action has focused around the issue of repairs and maintenance of council housing. This is reflected in the literature. The Association of Community Workers, for instance, devoted a publication to community work and tenant action (Henderson et al., 1982), and considerable space was allocated to housing-related issues in the now defunct magazine *Community Action*.

An important strand of community action has been that linked with trade union activity (see, for example, Corkey and Craig, 1978; Craig et al., 1979). This has often been as a direct result of the work of the Community Development Projects in a particular locality. Examples of the projects that arose from such an intervention include the Coventry Workshop, the Tyneside Trade Union Studies Unit, and the Joint Docklands Action Group. This type of action has been further developed in the 1980s and 1990s by municipal socialism, which has been based on a broad political group described as the 'new urban left.' Towards the end of the existence of the Greater London Council there were a plethora of supported community projects. However, Goodwin and Duncan (1986) argue that such policies are most effective in terms of political mobilization and that policy-makers on the left should be aware of the constraints and limitations of policies promising large-scale job creation and local economic regeneration. With rising unemployment, the issue of community action and the problems faced by people without employment became a concern during the early 1980s and have continued to be so to the present day (Cumella, 1984; Gallacher et al., 1983; McMichael et al., 1990; Ohri and Roberts, 1981; Purcell, 1982; Salmon, 1984), while community action and co-operatives have also been an important theme (*Roof*, 1986).

The role of the community worker in the community action model is an interesting one and highlights the tension within the state towards community work. We have noted in previous discussions that the majority of community work is sponsored by the state, which, through its agencies, will define, supervise and regulate the work of practitioners. However, community action, by its very nature, is often engaged in conflict with the employers of community workers, the local authorities. A wider debate on the contradictions surrounding this position is addressed in *In and Against the State* (London Edinburgh Weekend Return Group, 1980). It is for this reason that community action is usually seen as an area of practice undertaken by campaigners and activists who are not employed, directly or indirectly, by the state. Thomas (1983) argues that one cannot conflate the role of community worker with that of community activist. They are, in his view, different, and clearly reflect his own adherence to the pluralist approach and practice theories.

> Community work interventions require a certain degree of experience and training; they offer specific skills and knowledge to a community or agency which are different from (although not inherently better than and often over lapping with) those offered by local residents who take on active roles within community groups. (Thomas, 1983: 11)

In the same book, which reviews the development of community work, Thomas does not discuss the role of community action other than in passing reference. Instead he focuses on community work as a specialist occupation, with 'a particular and limited intervention' (Thomas, 1983: 7), located in neighbourhoods and agencies. The decision by Thomas not to address the community action model highlights his view that community work is a profession, rather than a political activity.

FEMINIST COMMUNITY WORK

Feminist community work theory evolved based on the development, since the 1960s, of feminist theory. Female community workers have applied these theoretical understandings to practice (see, for example, Dixon et al., 1982), both in feminist campaigns and in permeating existing community work practice and principles (Dominelli, 1994; Dominelli and McLeod, 1989). While there is no agreed single theoretical feminist position, there is a consensus that the central aim of feminist community work practice is the improvement of women's welfare by collectively challenging the social determinants of women's inequality. Although much of the practice is focused at the personal, local or neighbourhood level, it is linked practically and theoretically with wider feminist concerns. For example, women have been active in many localities in providing accommodation, usually in the form of emergency housing, for battered women. This securement of safe accommodation is a response to the immediate suffering experienced by individual women at the hands of violent men, as well as presenting a stand against male violence (see, for example, Binney et al., 1981; Hanmer and Maynard, 1987; Pahl, 1985a; Wilson, 1983).

The women's movement has had a central role as a feature of new social movements. Feminist campaigns are an example of practice that links local work with that undertaken at national level. As well as the example of local women's refuges, which are affiliated to the National Women's Aid Federation, we can note a number of other campaigns and networks which have both a local and a national profile. These include women's health groups (Roberts, 1982; Ruzek, 1986; Webb, 1986); women's involvement in the 1984-5 miners' strike (Bloomfield, 1986; Dolby, 1987; Lewycka, 1986; McCrindle and Rowbotham, 1986; Millar, 1987; Seddon, 1986; Waddington et al., 1991; Whitham, 1986); the National

Childcare Campaign, which while influenced by the women's movement, included fathers, trade union members and social services workers (NCC, 1985); the Programme of the Reform on the Law of Soliciting (PROS), a Birmingham based group of prostitutes whose aim was the abolition of prison sentences for loitering and soliciting (McLeod, 1982); the Wages for Housework grouping (Malos, 1980), the National Houseworking Group (Allen and Wolkowitz, 1986), and the Leicester Outwork Campaign (1987); abortion campaigns (Berer, 1988); campaigns highlighting the link between pornography and violence (Segal, 1990); Rape Crisis Centres (Pahl, 1985b); women's therapy centres (Doyal and Elston, 1986); Incest Survivor Groups (Armstrong, 1987; Dominelli, 1986, 1989; Kelly, 1988); the revolutionary feminist initiative Women Against Violence Against Women (McNeil and Rhodes, 1985); and the women's peace movement, in particular that focused on Greenham Common (Cook and Kirk, 1983; Feminism and Non-Violence Study Group, 1983; Finch, 1986; Harford and Hopkins, 1984). 'Women's issues' were also incorporated into developments in municipal socialism, but not without a degree of resistance from men (Cockburn, 1991).

As well as the commitment to working collectively to challenge and eradicate inequalities suffered by women, feminist community work practice emphasizes the objective of working with women's own personal experiences in groups. According to one influential writer in this area, this helps

> redefine social problems and challenges the individualising and pathologising approaches to women's issues marking the practice of traditional community workers and social workers. Crucial to this challenge has been undoing the division of social problems into private matters requiring individual or family solutions and public issues in which a range of social forces including the state, formal agencies and the public intervened. (Dominelli, 1990, 43)

This work is often undertaken in the form of consciousness-raising groups. Women's consciousness-raising groups are intended to break down feelings of isolation and provide participants with a sense of solidarity in order to engage in co-operative struggles. As we have seen above, consciousness-raising groups can also provide women with the strength, knowledge and skill to challenge professionals' definition of their positions. Overall, these groups are considered by feminist community workers as an important first step in the process of change; it is a necessary but not sufficient condition for the transformation of social relations.

The use of women only groups, whether in specialist consciousness raising or in more general ways, is a central feature of feminist community work. Among its advocates, Hanmer and Statham (1988) argue that the quality of the group process is likely to be improved in a single-sex group, because the intimate and interpersonal problems are likely to be confronted more quickly. The authors claim that the realization that their problems are not unique should help to reduce women's feelings of personal inadequacy, and thus start to alleviate isolation and stigmatization. Similarly, research has shown that men take over and influence community groups by controlling the 'introduction and pursuit of topics, the use of available time, the lack of emotional content in conversation' (Hanmer and Statham, 1988, 131). This is confirmed by Gallacher (1977), who notes that men hold key positions in community associations.

Feminist community workers have engaged in a variety of creative attempts to develop non-hierarchical structures and more participatory ways of working. Criticisms of traditional forms of organization as being alienating and inaccessible initially resulted in attempts to develop structureless groups. However, there is a recognition that it is 'a mistake to equate structure with hierarchy' (Freeman, 1984: 62). This has led one writer to argue that 'the quest for a structure which is genuinely participatory, which does not alienate people, and yet achieves the goals which the group has set itself must be central to feminist practice within the women's movement and in community work' (Barker, 1986: 87).

Similarly, process models in group work have been of concern to feminist community workers who indicate that they can function to exclude and to intimidate group members. Process models are concerned with both the different stages a group moves through (for instance, reflection, planning and action) and the development individual group members achieve. According to Brown (1986), process models have two ideologically different positions. One emphasizes individual emotional growth and development. The model is founded upon political and social philosophies and is engaged in achieving change for disadvantaged people. Previously the importance of process has been overlooked by radical community work because of the dominance of the former model. Dixon et al. (1982) argue, for instance, that this non-political approach was reflected in the writings of early theorists such as Batten. However, as they go on to state, 'Feminist analysis shows clearly that process is political, and needs urgent consideration if our campaigns are to achieve their aims' (Dixon et al., 1982: L 63).

The concern with regard to feminist community work is that the flow of written work in this area has been reduced to a trickle. The lack of recent feminist community work literature is commented upon by Dominelli (1990: 8), who highlights the fact that two of the main exponents of community work literature, David Thomas and Alan Twelvetrees, have 'virtually ignored the implications of gender.' Similarly, more radical texts appear to have included little on gender, something noted by Brandwein (1987) and Lee and Weeks (1991). When one considers the role women play in community work, whether as activists as described by Campbell (1993), or in administering a community work project as discussed by Brandwein (1987), it is clear that women have played a highly significant part in the practice. Dominelli (1990: 122) argues that women's contribution to community work has been undervalued. For instance, while there are texts that track the campaign work women have been engaged in (see Curno et al., 1982; Mayo, 1977), the perception of women themselves has rarely been considered. The paucity of literature in this field indicates the need for further research and dissemination of results, if we are to increase our understanding in this important sphere of community work.

BLACK AND ANTI-RACIST COMMUNITY WORK

Traditional forms of community work have failed both to meet the particular needs of the black community[1] and to challenge institutional and personal racism. There is considerable response to this problem from the black community and those community workers who are engaged in developing an anti-racist critique.

Historically there is evidence that the black community has not passively accepted racism and racist policy and practice. Since their arrival in Britain, black people have been active in their communities, supporting each other and organizing to resist discrimination and defend their rights (Bhat et al., 1988; Hiro, 1992; Solomos, 1989). The focus of discrimination has varied, although frequently it has appeared as if black people have been and continue to be besieged in a number of areas including education, housing, immigration, health, employment, and police relations. Similarly, a range of different and overlapping responses has developed: campaigns; self-help groups; direct action; alternative and supplementary provision. At times these have required coalitions to be built and alliances forged, at others autonomous organization has been preferred. Unfortunately, for our purposes, few studies have been made of these community-based organizations and campaigns. At the time of writing, a detailed survey of the nature of black voluntary groups, their activities, sources and level of funding, composition and organization, is being undertaken by the Organization Development Unit of the National Council for Voluntary Organisations. Those studies that have been made tend to be limited in their scope (Solomos, 1989: 149). There is also evidence of black people being excluded from mainstream political life in Britain, which has led to migrants launching a number of local and national groupings including the Indian Workers' Association and the West Indian Standing Conference (Carter, 1986; Jacobs, 1986). Furthermore, Anwar (1986) argues that racial disadvantage and discrimination will only be solved when black people are included in the political process and in British public life.

The studies that have been made of the influence of black community-based organizations and groups provide useful insights. For instance, the work by Goulbourne (1987, 1990) indicates that certain autonomous black community-based groups have successfully influenced mainstream institutions by placing on the political agenda contentious issues, such as police relations with the black community and the education of black children. Cheetham (1988) meanwhile argues that ethnic associations in Britain have a vitality and energy that has assisted their development as active self-help groups. Kalka (1991) discusses the tension between entrenched local organizations and newly founded ethnic associations and pressure groups. The author describes the situation in the London Borough of Harrow where Gujarati Hindus became increasingly articulate in presenting demands and acquiring new skills to assert their position. Not all black groups have been able to gain effective representation and satisfactory resources. Bangladeshis are thought to be disadvantaged relative to other Asian communities in Britain (Carey and Shukur, 1985-86), while according to Fawzi El-Solh (1991) Somalis living in the Tower Hamlets area of London's East End, who rank as one of the oldest settled migrant groups in Britain's docklands, experience greater difficulties. Fawzi El-Solh argues that Somalis encounter obstacles to effective organization of their community, while their needs are not satisfactorily represented.

Other research that describes and discusses the role of, and work with, black community-based groups includes that by Sondhi (1982). Writing about his work at the Asian Resource Centre in the multi-racial community of Handsworth in Birmingham, Sondhi views the agency as a campaigning one that provides a much needed advice and information service in the locality. The agency also undertook specific work with the Asian elderly (Asian Sheltered Residential Accommodation, 1981). Mullard (1973) argues, however, that state-supported self-help groups channel the energy of black militants away from wider political struggles. This view is supported by James (1990), who believes that politically motivated and articulate black professionals suffer from a constant tension centered on the issue of whom they can best serve. In many cases such professionals have been absorbed into local authorities' hierarchies or into academic posts, and in the process have modified, or have been required to modify, their demands for improvements in the position of the black community. At the same time such workers retain their loyalty and commitment to their own community. This leads to black workers experiencing burnout, frustration and anger. On the one hand they are

> actively working with policy makers and colleagues to address the issues. On the other spending evenings and weekends with

> volunteers and community activists to help them articulate about the issues so that they may eventually work with the policy makers. (James, 1990, 32)

The establishment of community projects by the black population is often a response to exclusion from white-dominated provision as well as providing opportunities to develop and strengthen cultural, social and political ties. Although black people do not form a homogeneous group within Britain, they share with each other the experience of racism and of colonization which, as we noted earlier, has given them certain strengths and perspectives. Community work projects funded by the Commission for Racial Equality and Racial Equality Council, have, however, met with criticism from two different sources. One argues that public funds should be given to projects that are for the whole community and not one particular group. This argument fails, however, to recognize structural racism, which leads to black people being excluded from mainstream organizations and the need for them to have separate provision. The other source of criticism has come from black radicals such as Sivanandan (1976: 1990), who believes that such projects dissolve and co-opt black protest. Within white-dominated community work the activity has only gradually addressed the issue of racism and it is felt in a number of quarters this has only been partial (Dominelli, 1990; Ohri et al., 1982). According to one writer, the central issue that needs to be addressed by white community workers is the continuing failure of institutions to provide equal treatment of black people while recognizing the specific needs of ethnic minorities (Loney, 1983: 54).

On a wider level, since the passing of the 1948 British Nationality Act, and up to and since the 1988 Immigration Act, 'race' and immigration have been central issues in British political life. During the early 1980s a number of mainly Labour-controlled local authorities attempted to operate and implement racial equality policies and practices. In at least one study these were to prove that the local political scene was an important site of struggle, particularly for local organizations committed to racial equality (Ben-Tovim et al., 1986). The abolition of the Greater London Council in March 1986 was believed to have serious implications for black residents of the capital since it left no city-wide commitment to support the black community and no agreement to tackle racism (Adeyemi, 1985). There has been some criticism by black writers that well-intentioned white people incorporated the black struggle in the local authority anti-racist strategies of this period (see, for example, Bhavnani, 1986; Gilroy, 1987). These writers and others (Mullard, 1984; Troyna, 1987; Troyna and Carrington, 1990) criticize multicultural education strategies which emphasize cultural pluralism and equality in a setting of economic and social inequality. With these limitations recognized, it is important not to overlook the contribution from white anti-racists in community work to the struggle for equal opportunities and for the provision for more resources for the black community, and in 'confront[ing] racism, sexism and other forms of discrimination both within ourselves and within society' (Association of Community Workers, 1982).

An example of community workers with an anti-racist approach successfully confronting racism and harassment is offered by Buckingham and Martin (1989). Working in and around a north London housing estate, the workers describe and reflect on their use of community development principles and practice to reduce the harassment endured by the Bangladeshis living in the area. A further example is a training aid for confronting anti-racism in the form of a video that has been produced by Rooney Martin (1987). The video shows a group of white people from a variety of backgrounds including English, Irish, Jewish and working-class, discussing what it means to be white from their particular standpoint. The main function of the video is to sensitize white people to the need to understand whiteness and how their colour affects their culture and their relationships with non-white people.

The national Commission for Racial Equality and local Racial Equality Councils have been active in supporting black and anti-racist community work. The national survey by Francis et al. (1984: 11) found that 72% of all Community Relations Councils' community workers came from black groups, and whereas 59% of all community workers were employed in the voluntary sector, 81% of black community workers were employed in this sector. There have been certain criticisms, however, that the black community should not have to rely on government-sponsored bodies or the voluntary sector, but rather they need to be able to deal directly with their local authorities and elected representatives. John (1981) argues, for instance, that black workers should be employed by local authorities rather than by a vulnerable, often unaccountable voluntary sector which serves to place the needs of the black community at the margins of social and political life.

Finally, Ohri et al. (1982) argue that the primary issue for the black community and the one which community work must address if it is to remain relevant to the needs and concerns of black people, is the resistance to racism.

CONCLUSION

In conclusion, we can see that although there is overlap between the models discussed, particularly in terms of techniques and skills used, the models reflect different traditions and ideologies. Community care, community organization, community development and social/community planning represent the pluralist tradition in community work. The community action model and the emerging models from feminism and the black and anti-racist critique reflect a radical and socialist approach. Different aspects of community education fit into different approaches. The radical strand of the model is epitomized in the work of Freire and of Lovett. The work of school-based community education, including the compensatory education programmes, is, however, an example of the pluralist approach. Certain models, for instance community care and social/community planning, are centered upon the premise of delivering a service in a more efficient and often cost-effective or cost-saving manner. Other models, such as those from the radical and socialist approaches, are focused around certain ideological positions and commitments. Together with the remaining models the above offers us a framework in which to understand community work practice.

NOTE

1. In the United Kingdom, the term "black" refers to populations of African, Asian, and Indian descent.

REFERENCES

Adamson, N., Briskin, L. and McPhail, M. (1988). *Organizing for Change: The Contemporary Women's Movement in Canada.* Oxford: Oxford University Press.

Adeyemi, F. (1985). "The Abolition of the G.L.C.: The Implications for the Black Community," *Talking Point*, no. 65. Newcastle upon Tyne: Association of Community Workers.

Alinsky, S. (1969). *Reveille for Radicals.* New York: Vintage Books.

Alinsky, S. (1971). *Rules for Radicals.* New York: Random House.

Allen, G., Bastiani, J., Martin, I. and Richards, K. (eds.) (1987). *Community Education: An Agenda for Educational Reform.* Milton Keynes: Open University Press.

Allen, S. and Wolkowitz, C. (1986). "The Control of Women's Labour: The Case of Homeworking," *Feminist Review* 22, Spring: 25-51.

Allman, P. (1987). "Paulo Freire's Education: A Struggle for Meaning: in Allen, G., Bastiani, J., and Martin, I. (eds.), *Community Education: An Agenda for Educational Reform.* Milton Keynes: Open University Press.

Anionwu, E. (1990). "Community Development Approaches to Sickle Cell Anaemia," *Talking Point*, no. 113. Newcastle upon Tyne: Association of Community Workers.

Anwar, M. (1986). *Race and Politics, Ethnic Minorities and the British Political System.* London: Tavistock.

Armstrong, L. (1987). *Kiss Daddy Goodnight.* New York: Random House.

Asian Sheltered Residential Accommodation (1981). *Asian Sheltered Residential Accommodation.* London: Asian Sheltered Residential Accommodation.

Association of Community Workers (1982). *ACW Definition of Community Work.* London: Association of Community Workers.

Barclay, P. M. (1982). *Social Workers: Their Role and Tasks (The Barclay Report).* London: Bedford Square Press.

Barker, H. (1986). "Recapturing Sisterhood: A Critical Look at "Process" in Feminist Organising and Community Work," *Critical Social Policy*, 16, Summer: 80-90.

Barr, A. (1991). *Practising Community Development: Experience in Strathclyde.* London: Community Development Foundation.

Batten, T. R. (1957). *Communities and Their Development.* London: Oxford University Press.

Batten, T. R. (1962). *Training for Community Development: A Critical Study of Method.* London: Oxford University Press.

Batten, T. R. (1965). *The Human Factor in Community Work.* London: Oxford University Press.

Batten, T. R., with the collaboration of Madge Batten (1967). *The Non-directive Approach in Group and Community Work.* London: Oxford University Press.

Ben-Tovim, G., Gabriel, J., Law, I. and Stedder, K. (1986). *The Local Politics of Race.* London: Macmillan.

Berer, M. (1988). "Whatever Happened to A Women's Right to Choose?", *Feminist Review*, 29, Spring: 24-37.

Beresford, P. and Croft, S. (1986). *Whose Welfare? Private Care or Public Services.* Brighton: The Lewis Cohen Urban Studies Centre at Brighton Polytechnic.

Bhat, A., Carr-Hill, R. and Ohri, S. (eds.) (1988). *Britain's Black Population: A New Perspective* (2nd edn). Aldershot: Gower.

Bhavnani, R. (1986). "The Struggle for an Anti-Racist Policy in Education in Avon," *Critical Social Policy*, 16: 104-8.

Biddle L., and Biddle, W. (1965). *The Community Development Process: The Rediscovery of Local Initiative*. New York: Holt, Rinehart & Winston.

Binney, V., Harkell, G. and Nixon, J. (1981). *Leaving Violent Men: A Study of Refugees and Housing for Battered Women*. London: Women's Aid Federation.

Bloomfield, B. (1986). "Women's Support Groups at Maerdy" in Samuel, R., Bloomfield, B. and Boanas, G. (eds.), *The Enemy Within: Pit Villages and the Miners Strike of 1984-5*. London: Routledge & Kegan Paul.

Brandwein, R. A. (1987). "Women and Community Organisation" in Burden, D. S. and Gottlieb, N. (eds.), *The Woman Client*. London: Tavistock.

Brown, A. (1986). *Groupwork*. London: Heinemann Educational Books.

Buckingham, G. and Martin, M. (1989). "Community Development, Harassment and Racism," *Talking Point*, no. 103. Newcastle upon Tyne: Association of Community Workers.

CDP (1977). *Gilding the Ghetto: The State and The Poverty Experiments*. London: Community Development Project Inter-project Editorial Team.

Campbell, B. (1993). "Stand of a Local Heroine," *Guardian*, 25, January.

Carey, S. and Shukur, A. (1985-6). "A Profile of the Bangladeshi Community in East London," *New Community*, 12(3): 405-17.

Carter, T. (1986). *Shattering Illusions*. London: Lawrence and Wishart.

Cheetham, J. (1988). "Ethnic Associations in Britain" in Jenkins, S. (ed.), *Ethnic Associations and the Welfare State*. New York: Columbia University Press.

Cockburn, C. (1977). *The Local State*. London: Pluto Press.

Cockburn, C. (1991). *In the Way of Women: Men's Resistance to Sex Equality in Organizations*. Basingstoke: Macmillan.

Cook, A. and Kirk, G. (1983). *Greenham Women Everywhere: Dreams, Ideas and Action from the Women's Peace Movement*. London: Pluto Press.

Corkey, D. and Craig, G. (1978). "Community Work or Class Politics?" in Curno, P. (ed.), *Political Issues and Community Work*. London: Routledge & Kegan Paul.

Cowley, J., Kaye, A., Mayo, M. and Thompson, M. (1977). *Community or Class Struggle*. London: Stage 1.

Craig, G., Mayo, M. and Sharman, N. (1979). *Jobs and Community Action: Community Work Five*. London: Routledge & Kegan Paul in association with the Association of Community Workers.

Craig, G., Derricourt, N. and Loney, M. (eds.) (1982). *Community Work and the State: Towards a Radical Practice: Community Work Eight*. London: Routledge & Kegan Paul in association with the Association of Community Workers.

Croft, S. (1986). "Women, Caring and the Recasting of Need," *Critical Social Policy*, 16: 23-39.

Cumella, M. (1984). "Community Work and Unemployment-The Aftermath of the "Slimline" of the Steel Industry in Newport, South Wales," COMM 22, August. Marcinelle, Belgium: Inter-University European Institute of Social Welfare, rue du Debarcadere, 179, B-6001 Marcinelle.

Curno, A., Lamming, A., Leach, L., Stiles, J., Ward, V. and Ziff, T. (1982). *Women in Collective Action*. Newcastle upon Tyne: Association of Community Workers.

Curno , P. (ed.) (1978). *Political Issues and Community Work: Community Work Four*. London: Routledge & Kegan Paul.

DES (1967). *Children and Their Primary Schools*. Report to the Central Advisory Council for Education, No. 1 (Plowden Report). London: HMSO.

Dalley, G. (1988). *Ideologies of Caring: Rethinking Community and Collectivism*. London: Macmillan.

Dearlove, J. (1974). "The Control of Change and the Regulations of Community Action" in Jones, D. and Mayo, M. (eds.) *Community Work One*. London: Routledge and Kegan Paul.

Dixon, G., Johnson, C., Leigh, S. and Turnbull, N. (1982). "Feminist Perspectives and Practice" in Craig, G., Derricourt, N. and Loney, M. (eds.), *Community Work and the State: Towards a Radical Practice: Community Work Eight*. London: Routledge and Kegan Paul.

Dolby, N. (1987). *Norma Dolby's Diary*. London: Verso.

Dominelli, L. (1986). "Father-Daughter Incest: Patriarchy's Shameful Secret," *Critical Social Policy*, 16: 8-22.

Dominelli, L. (1989). "Betrayal of Trust: A Feminist Analysis of Power Relationships in Incest Abuse," *British Journal of Social Work*, 19(4): 291-302.

Dominelli, L. (1990). *Women and Community Action*. Birmingham: Venture Press.

Dominelli, L. (1994). "Women, Community Work and the State in the 1990s" in Jacobs, S. and Popple, K. (eds.), *Community Work in the 1990s*. Nottingham: Spokesman.

Dominelli, L. and McLeod, E. (1989). *Feminist Social Work*. London: Macmillan.

Doyal, L. and Elston, M. A. (1986). "Women, Health and Medicine" in Beechey, V. and Whitelegg, E. (eds.), *Women in Britain Today*. Milton Keynes: Open University Press.

Equal Opportunities Commission (1984). *Carers and Services: A Comparison of Men and Women Caring for Dependent Elderly People*. Manchester: Equal Opportunities Commission.

Fairbairn, A. (1979). *The Leicestershire Community Colleges and Centres*. Nottingham: Nottingham University/National Institute for Adult Education.

Family Policy Studies Centre (1989). *Family Policy Bulletin*, no. 6. London: Family Policy Studies Centre.

Fawzi El-Solh, C. (1991). "Somalis in London's East End: A Community Striving for Recognition," *New Community*, 17(4): 539-52.

Feminism and Non-Violence Study Group (1983). *Piecing it Together: Feminism and Non-violence*. Buckleigh: Feminism and Non-Violence Group.

Finch, J. (1984). "Community Care: Developing Non-sexist Alternatives," *Critical Social Policy*, 9: 6-18.

Finch, J. and Groves, D. (eds.) (1983). *A Labour of Love: Women, Work and Caring*. London: Routledge & Kegan Paul.

Finch, J. and Groves, D. (1985). "Community Care and the Family: A Case for Equal Opportunities" in Ungerson, C. (ed.), *Women and Social Policy: A Reader*. London: Macmillan.

Finch, S., with Mary, Cynthia, Linda, Colleen, Barbara and Jan, from Hackney Greenham Group (1986). "Socialist Feminism and Greenham," *Feminist Review*, 23, Summer: 93-100.

Foucault, M. (1967). *Madness and Civilisation: A History of Insanity*. London: Tavistock.

Foucault, M. (1977). *Discipline and Punishment: The Birth of Prison*. Harmondsworth: Allen Lane.

Francis, D., Henderson, P. and Thomas, D. N. (1984). *A Survey of Community Workers in the United Kingdom*. London: National Institute for Social Work.

Freeman, J. (1984). *The Tyranny of Structurelessness*. London: Dark Star and Rebel Press.

Freire, P. (1970). *Cultural Action for Freedom*. Harmondsworth: Penguin.

Freire, P. (1972). *Pedagogy of the Oppressed*. Harmondsworth: Penguin.

Freire, P. (1976). *Education: The Practice of Freedom*. London: Writers and Readers Publishing Cooperative.

Freire, P. (1985). *The Politics of Education: Culture, Power and Liberation*. London: Macmillan.

Gallacher, A. (1977). "Women and Community Work" in Mayo, M. (ed.), *Women in the Community*. London: Routledge & Kegan Paul in association with Association of Community Workers.

Gilroy, P. (1987). *There Ain't No Black in the Union Jack. The Cultural Politics of Race and Nation*. London: Hutchinson.

Goffman, E. (1961). *Asylums*. New York: Doubleday.

Goodwin, M. and Duncan, S. (1986). "The Local State and Local Economic Policy: Political Mobilisation or Economic Regeneration" in *Capital and Class*, 27, Winter: 14-36.

Goulbourne, H. (1987). "West Indian Groups and British Politics," paper presented to the Conference on Black People and British Politics, University of Warwick, November.

Goulbourne, H. D. (ed.) (1990). *Black Politics in Britain*. Aldershot: Avebury.

Griffiths, Sir Roy (1988). *Community Care: Agenda for Action*. London: HMSO.

HMSO (1954). *Social Development in the British Colonial Territories*. Report of the Ashbridge Conference on Social Development (Colonial Office), 3-12 August. London: HMSO.

HM Treasury (1987). *Treasury Report*. London: HMSO.

Hadley, R. and Hatch, S. (1981). *Social Welfare and the Failure of the State: Centralised Social Services and Participation*. London: Allen & Unwin.

Hadley, R. and McGrath, M. (1980). *Going Local: Neighbourhood and Social Services*. London: Bedford Square Press.

Hadley, R., Cooper, M., Dale, P. and Stacey, G. (1987). *A Community Social Worker's Handbook*. London: Tavistock.

Halsey, A. H. (ed.) (1972). *Educational Priority*. London: HMSO.

Hanmer, J. and Maynard, M. (1987). *Women, Violence and Social Control*. Basingstoke: Macmillan.

Hanmer, J. and Statham, D. (1988). *Women and Social Work: Towards a Woman-Centered Practice*. Basingstoke: Macmillan.

Harford, B. and Hopkins, S. (eds.) (1984). *Greenham Common: Women and the Wire*. London: Women's Press.

Heginbotham, C. (1990). *Return to the Community: The Voluntary Ethic and Community Care*. London: Bedford Square Press.

Henderson, P., Wright, A. and Wyncoll, K. (eds.) (1982). *Successes and Struggles on Council Estates: Tenant Action and Community Work*. London: Association of Community Workers.

Hiro, D. (1992). *Black British, White British: A History of Race Relations in Britain*. London: Paladin.

Jacobs, B. (1986). *Black Politics and the Urban Crisis in Britain*. Cambridge: Cambridge University Press.

James, J. (1990). "Public Services and the Black Community" in Schofield, A. (ed.), *Report of the Social Work Education and Racism Workshop 29th-30th March 1990 at Ruskin College*. Oxford: Community Education Research and Training Unit, Ruskin College.

John, G. (1981). *In the Service of Black Youth: The Political Culture of Youth and Community Work with Black People in English Cities*. Leicester: National Association of Youth Clubs.

Jones, D. (1977). "Community Work in the United Kingdom" in Specht, H. and Vickery, A. (eds.), *Integrating Social Work Methods*. London: Allen & Unwin.

Jones, D. and Mayo, M. (eds.) (1975). *Community Work Two*. London: Routledge & Kegan Paul.

Jones, K. and Fowles, A. J. (1984). *Ideas on Institutions*. London: Routledge & Kegan Paul.

Kalka, I. (1991). "The Politics of the "Community" among Gujarati Hindus in London," *New Community*, 17(3): 377-85.

Kelly, L. (1988). *Surviving Sexual Violence*. Cambridge: Polity Press.

Kramer, R. (1979). "Voluntary Agencies in the Welfare State: An Analysis of the Vanguard Role," *Journal of Social Policy*, 8(4): 473-88.

Lamoureux, H., Mayer, R. and Panet-Raymond, J. (1989). *Community Action*. Quebec: Black Rose Books.

Lapping, A. (ed.) (1970). *Community Action* (Fabian Tract 400). London: Fabian Society.

Leavitas, R. (ed.) (1986). *The Ideology of the New Right*. Cambridge: Polity Press.

Lee, B. and Weeks, W. (1991). "Social Action Theory and the Women's Movement: An Analysis of Assumption," *Community Development Journal*, 26(3): 220-26.

Lees, R. and Mayo, M. (1984). *Community Action for Change*. London: Routledge & Kegan Paul.

Leicester Outwork Campaign (1987). *Leicester Outwork Campaign Annual Report* 1986-87. Leicester: Leicester Outwork Campaign, 132 Regent Road, Leicester LE1 7PA.

Leonard, P. (ed.) (1975). *The Sociology of Community Action*, Sociological Review Monograph 21. Keele: University of Keele.

Lewis, J. and Meredith, B. (1990). *Daughters Who Care*. London: Routledge.

Lewycka, M. (1986). "The Way They Were," *New Socialist*, 36, March: 16-18.

London Edinburgh Weekend Return Group (1980). *In and Against the State*. London: Pluto Press.

Loney, M. (1983). *Community against Government: The British Community Development Project* 1968-78. London: Heinemann Educational Books.

Loney, M., Bocock, R., Clarke, J., Cochrane, A., Graham, P. and Wilson, M. (eds.) (1991). *The State or the Market: Politics Welfare in Contemporary Britain* (Second Edition). London: Sage in association with Open University Press.

Lovett, T. (1975). *Adult Education, Community Development and the Working Class*. London: Ward Lock.

Lovett, T., Clarke, C. and Kilmurray, A. (1983). *Adult Education and Community Action*. London: Croom Helm.

McCrindle, J., and Rowbotham, S. (1986). "More Than Just a Memory," *Feminist Review*, 23, Summer: 109-24.

McLeod, E. (1982). *Women Working: Prostitution Now*. London: Croom Helm.

McMichael, P., Lynch, B. and Wright, D. (1990). *Building Bridges into Work: The Role of the Community Worker*. Harlow: Longman.

McNeil, S. and Rhodes, D. (eds.) (1985). *Women Against Violence against Women*. London: Only Women Press.

Malos, E. (1980). *The Politics of Housework*. London: Allen & Busby.

Marris, P. (1987). *Meaning and Action: Planning and Conceptions of Change*. London: Routledge & Kegan Paul.

Martin, I. (1987). "Community Education: Towards a Theoretical Analysis" in Allen, G., Bastiani, J., Martin, I. and Richards, K. (eds.), *Community Education: An Agenda for Educational Reform*. Milton Keynes: Open University Press.

Mayo, M. (ed.) (1977). *Women in the Community. Community Work Three*. London: Routledge & Kegan Paul.

Mayo, M. (1980). "Beyond CDP: reaction and community action" in Bailey, R. and Brake, M. (eds.), *Radical Social Work and Practice*. London: Edward Arnold.

Mayo, M. (1982). "Community Action Programmes in the Early Eighties-What Future?", *Critical Social Policy*, 1(3): 5-18.

Mayo, M. and Jones, D. (eds.) (1974). *Community Work One*. London: Routledge & Kegan Paul.

Midwinter, E. (1972). *Priority Education*. Harmondsworth: Penguin.

Midwinter, E. (1975). *Education and the Community*. London: George Allen & Unwin.

Millar, J. (1987). *You Can't Kill the Spirit*. London: Women's Press.

Morris, H. (1925). *The Village College: Being a Memorandum on the Provision of Educational and Social Facilities for the Countryside, with Special Reference to Cambridgeshire*. Cambridge: Cambridge University Press.

Morris, J. (1990). *Pride Without Prejudice*. London: Women's Press.

Morris, P. (1969). *Put Away: A Sociological Study of Institutions for the Mentally Retarded*. London: Routledge & Kegan Paul.

Mullard, C. (1973). *Black Britain*. London: Allen & Unwin.

Mullard, C. (1984). *Anti-Racist Education: The Three O's*. Cardiff: National Anti-racist Movement in Education.

National Child Care Campaign (1985). *National Childcare Campaign Policy Statement*. London: National Child Care Campaign.

Newham Docklands Forum and Greater London Council Popular Planning Unit (1983). *People's Plan for the Royal Docks*. London: Greater London Council.

Ng, R. (1988). *The Politics of Community Services: Immigrant Women, Class and the State*. Toronto: Garamond Press.

Ohri, A., Manning, B. and Curno, P. (eds.) (1982). *Community Work and Racism: Community Work Seven*. London: Routledge & Kegan Paul in association with the Association of Community Workers.

Ohri, A. and Roberts, L. (1981). "Can Community Workers Do Anything about Unemployment?", *Talking Point*, no. 28. London: Association of Community Workers.

O'Malley, J. (1977). *Politics of Community Action*. London: Russell.

Pahl, J. (ed.) (1985a). *Private Violence and Public Policy: The Needs of Battered Women and the Response of the Public Services*. London: Routledge & Kegan Paul.

Pahl, J. (1985b). "Refuges for Battered Women: Ideology and Action," *Feminist Review*, 19, Spring: 25-43.

Parker, R. A. (1981). "Tending and Social Policy" in Goldberg, E. M. and Hatch, S. (eds.), *A New Look at the Personal Social Services*. London: Policy Studies Institute.

Piven, F. and Cloward, R. (1977). *Poor People's Movement: Why They Succeed, How They Fail*. New York: Vintage Books.

Purcell, R. (1982). "Community Action and Real Work," *Talking Point*, No. 32. London: Association of Community Workers.

Radford, J. (1970). "From King Hill to the Squatting Association" in Lapping, A. (ed.), *Community Action* (Fabian Tract 400). London: Fabian Society.

Ree, H. (1973). *Educator Extraordinary: The Life and Achievements of Henry Morris*. London: Longman.

Ree, H. (1985). *The Henry Morris Collection*. Cambridge: Cambridge University Press.

Robb, B. (ed.) (1967). *Sans Everything: A Case to Answer*. London: Nelson.

Roberts, H. (ed.) (1982). *Women's Health Matters*. London: Routledge.

Roberts, L. (1992). "A Community Development Perspective on Community Care," *Talking Point*, no. 132. Newcastle upon Tyne: Association of Community Workers.

Rogers, V. (1994). "Feminist Work and Community Education" in Jacobs, S. and Popple, K. (eds.), *Community Work in the 1990s*. Nottingham: Spokesman.

Roof (1986). "The Penny Drops at Coin Street," March/April: 6-7.

Rothman, J. (1970). "Three Models of Community Organisation Practice" in Cox, F., Erlich, J., Rothman, J. and Tropman, J. (eds.), *Strategies of Community Organisation*. Itaska, IL: Peacock Publishing.

Ruzek, S. (1986). "Feminist Visions of Health: An International Perspective" in Mitchell, J. and Oakley, A. (eds.), *What is Feminism?* Oxford: Basil Blackwell.

Salmon, H. (1984). *Unemployment: The Two Nations*. London: Association of Community Workers.

Scull, A. T. (1977). *Decarceration: Community Treatment and the Deviant: A Radical View*. Englewood Cliffs, NJ: Prentice Hall.

Seddon, V. (1986). *The Cutting Edge: Women and the Pit Strike*. London: Lawrence & Wishart.

Segal, L. (1990). "Pornography and Violence: What the "Experts" Really Say," *Feminist Review*, 36, Autumn.

Silburn, R. (1971). "The Potential and Limitations of Community Action" in Bull, D. (ed.), *Family Poverty*. London: Duckworth & Co.

Sivanandan, A. (1990). *Communities of Resistance: Writings on Black Struggles for Socialism*. London: Verso.

Smith, L. and Jones, D. (eds.) (1981). *Deprivation, Participation and Communication Action. Community Work Six*. London: Routledge & Kegan Paul.

Solomos, J. (1989). *Black Youth, Racism and the State: The Politics of Ideology and Policy*. Cambridge: Cambridge University Press.

Sondhi, R. (1982). "The Asian Resource Centre" in Cheetham, J. (ed.). *Ethnicity and Social Work*. Oxford: Oxford University Press.

Thomas, D. N. (1983). *The Making of Community Work*. London: George Allen & Unwin.

Townsend, P. (1962). *The Last Refuge: A Survey of Residential Institutions and Homes for the Aged in England and Wales*. London: Routledge & Kegan Paul.

Troyna, B. (1987). "Beyond Multi-culturalism: Towards the Enactment of Anti-racist Education in Policy, Provision and Pedagogy," *Oxford Review of Education*, 13(3): 307-20.

Troyna, B. and Carrington, B. (1990). *Education, Racism and Reform*. London: Routledge.

Twelvetrees, A. (1991). *Community Work* (2nd edn). London: Macmillan.

United Nations (1959). *European Seminar on Community Development and Social Welfare in Urban Areas*. Geneva: United Nations.

Ungerson, C. (1987). *Policy is Personal*. London: Tavistock.

Waddington, D., Wykes, M. and Chritcher, C. (1991). *Split at the Seam? Community, Continuity and Change after the 1984-5 Coal Dispute*. Milton Keynes: Open University Press.

Wagner, G. (1988). *Residential Care: A Positive Choice*. London: National Institute for Social Work/HMSO.

Walker, A. (1989). "Community Care" in McCarthy, M. (ed.), *The New Politics of Welfare*. Basingstoke: Macmillan Education.

Webb, C. (ed.) (1986). *Feminist Practice in Women's Health Care*. Chichester: Wiley.

Whitman, J. (1986). *Hearts and Minds*. London: Canary Press.

Wicks, M. (1987). *A Future for All*. Harmondsworth: Penguin.

Wilson, E. (1983). "Feminism and Social Policy" in Loney, M., Boswell, D. and Clarke, J. (eds.), *Social Policy and Social Welfare*. Milton Keynes: Open University Press.

Theory for Community Practice in Social Work: The Example of Ecological Community Practice

Ray H. MacNair, MSW, PhD

SUMMARY. The effort is made to revitalize the search for practice theory which will inform and guide the community practitioner. Ecological theory is used to identify a generic model of community practice and analyze member cohesion in the three traditional modalities. The theory of energy in human ecology is developed to set the stage for an energy assessment, and the selection of strategic energy patterns in phases of organizing. Theoretical propositions with practice implications are offered for research on the relationship between strategic energy-patterns of organizing, energy costs, specialization of function, and styles of intervention. *[Article copies available for a fee from The Haworth Document Delivery Service: 1-800-342-9678. E-mail address: getinfo@haworth.com]*

KEYWORDS. Community practice theory, ecological theory, social work practice, community organizing, community practice

---

Ray H. MacNair is Associate Professor of Social Work at the University of Georgia.

Address correspondence to: Ray H. MacNair, Associate Professor, School of Social Work, University of Georgia, Athens, GA 30602.

[Haworth co-indexing entry note]: "Theory for Community Practice in Social Work: The Example of Ecological Community Practice." MacNair, Ray H. Co-published simultaneously in *Journal of Community Practice* (The Haworth Press, Inc.) Vol. 3, No. 3/4, 1996, pp. 181-202; and: *Community Practice: Conceptual Models* (ed: Marie Weil) The Haworth Press, Inc., 1996, pp. 181-202. Single or multiple copies of this article are available for a fee from The Haworth Document Delivery Service [1-800-342-9678, 9:00 a.m. - 5:00 p.m. (EST). E-mail address: getinfo@haworth.com].

Scholars in the field of community practice are taking a renewed interest in the cumulative process of research and theory construction. This work arises from reflections on the recent three decades of history in the discipline. In 1963, Roland Warren first published his theoretical framework for community development, which he called the action system, within an analysis of communities. In the field of community practice theory, Warren established the social systems perspective (1963). This perspective has not been widely referenced by subsequent authors in the community organization field, nor have writers or teachers in the last twenty-eight years attempted systematically to construct an alternative theoretical framework. The unspoken assumption appears to be that theory is not relevant to the design of effective community organizing practices.

In the early 1970s, there was a brief flurry of theoretical activity focused on community practice (Rothman, 1974; Warren, 1974). Nevertheless, from the late 1970s through the 1980s, very little work was generated which could be employed by practitioners. In 1985, Taylor and Roberts concluded:

> Clearly, there is as yet no overarching theory of social work community practice. There are orientations and schools of thought, but the practitioner searching for a theory of community practice by which to guide and evaluate practice must still be patient. (p. 27)

The purpose of this paper is to contribute to a revitalization of theory development for community organization practice. A number of theoretical perspectives are available such as social exchange theory, role theory, and behavioral reinforcement theory, among others. This paper offers an illustration of the theory construction process in one area: applications of the overarching framework of ecological theory and the concept of human energy in community organizing to generate the concept of the ecological community practitioner.

ECOLOGICAL THEORY

An application of ecological theory to community organization practice begins with the biological analogy of ecological theory

(Hawley, 1950). This work posits individual organisms and species of organisms in an exchange relationship both with other organisms and with the natural elements within a specified environment. Ecological theory states that a balance of exchanges results in homeostasis, defined as a stabilization of habitats, functions, niches, and populations (Leiter & Webb, 1983). Conversely, unbalanced exchanges result in changes in the characteristics of populations, functions, and exchanges. For example, if a required nutrient, such as water, is suddenly absent within an organism's habitat, its population will probably dwindle and its byproducts will be less available to organisms which are dependent on those byproducts.

Human Ecology

Human ecology carries this analogy to human populations and human communities. It treats individuals, families, and organizations as units within a cluster of similar units which perform similar functions and occupy the same niche. Units which perform different functions are described as occupying a different niche. Both Germain (1985, 1991) and Leiter and Webb (1983) have pointed out that each individual, family, and organization must seek and negotiate the human and material resources it needs within its habitat, which is a community. These units symbiotically exchange their functions with units performing complementary functions, as in the case of a producer, grower, or developer exchanging their functions symbiotically with consumers. Another example is the clothing merchandiser exchanging resources with consumers whose money will be used to pay the merchandiser's staff who, in their turn, will purchase groceries. If each unit's function is to remain stable, a state of homeostasis must be reached among these exchanges. Material and uniquely human nutrients are also interdependent. It may be argued, for example, that a downturn in the economy which significantly reduces the ability of parents to provide for their children affects the emotional well-being of those parents, resulting in marital dissatisfaction and a withdrawal of the warm attentions that children need for their healthy development. Such imbalances, and the dysfunctional adaptations which result, do not lend themselves to such a simple explanation. The logic of such reverberations, however, over succeeding generations, is probably explanatory (Bronfenbrenner, 1986).

In ecological theory, interactions between economically functional adults, between parents, and between parents and children are not viewed in simple terms. Rather, they are seen as transactions in which the needs of the interacting parties are all taken into account. Germain (1985, p. 35) cites stress as one of the origins of adaptations of coping, which vary according to transactional competencies, a sense of self direction, relatedness to others, and self-esteem (personal efficacy):

> . . . adaptedness refers to the fit between persona in environment, the adaptive balance between needs, capacities, rights, and goals, and the qualities of the social and physical environment within a given culture. The fit is never fully achieved because people change and environments change, and each such change calls for further adaptations . . . adaptive processes include changes in the self to fit environmental pressures or opportunities; changes in the environment to make it fit human needs and requirements; or migration to new environments . . . adaption is a continuous process [involving] reciprocal shaping. . . .

The Ecology of Organizations

Human ecologists focus, among other things, on the web of organizations in a community that serve to sustain a population by negotiating resource exchanges and applying their expertise and coordinated human energies to some form of production, service, or trade activity. Symbiotic exchange makes sustenance possible for all functioning organizational units while they perform their specialized functions. Hence, symbiotic exchanges take place within the web of human service organizations through referrals while, at the same time, each organization exchanges functions with consumers to achieve their goals and, usually, some other source of funding in conjunction with consumers. Strategic planners, thinking ecologically, recognize immediately that changes in goals involve adaptations in the transactions with the resource environment for funding, consumers, and personnel.

Commensalism and Community Organizing

Hawley (1950, 1986) differentiates between symbiotic relationships, with complementary exchanges, and "commensalistic" relationships among people or organizations that perform the same or similar functions, called categoric units. Commensalism emerges within a perceived hostile, neglectful, or exploitive symbiotic environment. Mutual bonding among categoric units (who perform the same function) serves the purpose of gaining strength in such an environment.

An example of commensalism is labor unions which bond workers performing similar functions together. Typically, such workers identify with a common perception of management as exploitive. Civil rights organizations have been known to form coalitions when they determine that they will gain strength by working together in the face of a hostile, racist environment. Frequently, neighborhood organizations form federations, especially when they identify with similar socioeconomic lifestyles and residential objectives. Human service agencies band together in formal commensalistic organizations when they determine they could thereby strengthen the fund-raising capabilities of all their members, as in the case of United Way Agencies.

In principle, commensalism strengthens the bargaining power of categoric units which might otherwise compete with each other for scarce resources. One of the effects of commensalism is to conserve energy that would be devoted to competition among categoric units and save that energy for collective exchanges with the symbiotic environment.

In other words, commensalism is the antidote for a "divide and rule" strategy among corporate elites and policy makers. Individuals and families, experiencing similar frustrations, distress, and deprivation, may or may not collectively perceive the need for commensalistic bonding and mutual action. Indeed it may be those individuals most distressed and deprived who fail to develop the sense of efficacy required for collective action (Pecukonis & Wenocur, 1994). On the other hand, community practitioners do see the need and are challenged to generate the collective insight and interest needed for commensalistic organizing. The principles of commensalism are certainly the basis for most of community organization practice.

In summary, every unit within a community is involved in symbiotic exchanges. Every person, family, and organization performs a function, which others require, while receiving essential functions in return. The terms of the exchange may, however, be deemed fair and equitable, generating a healthy homeostasis, or they may be unfair and exploitive, resulting in the stress which produces either organized or dissipated reactions. By reducing competition among like units, however, commensalistic organizing conserves energy and makes it available for the exercise of power between the commensal organization and its symbiotic counterparts. The perception of a shared problem, the personal and collective sense of efficacy for organizing, and the discovery of the capabilities for organizing, among other things, contribute to the potential for cohesive commensalism and the promise of negotiating more equitable terms of sustenance.

THE GENERIC MODEL OF COMMUNITY PRACTICE IN ECOLOGICAL THEORY

Any community organization must draw its human and technical resources from its community environment, including categoric units and empathetic supporters who identify with their problems. In expending their human resources, participants expect to receive something in return, such as a reputation for power and improved living conditions for their constituency.

For the organization to be effective, however, its members must first understand the basis for their own commensalism. They must understand their common identity and their relation to environmental stresses (Germain, 1985). They must feel that their fair share is not achieved within the given terms of exchange. They must become aware of the availability of resources, controlled by others, which could be theirs. They must come to understand their own potential power with reference to the relative power of their targets. As internal cohesion becomes stronger and expression of needs becomes articulate, strategies of negotiation are more clearly designed, and campaign targets become more responsive.

Figure 1 below illustrates the Generic Ecological Model of community organizations and their practitioners within the community habitat. A community organization is organized, drawing its members from a constituency pool and its subjects. Through its constituency pool, it may draw strength from the functional sectors of the community: economic, governmental, educational, church and social club, and health and welfare institutions. The organizing process takes place, together with the catalytic guidance of a practitioner of community practice. An interventive strategy is selected, through which a target bureaucracy is approached for changes in policy or resources. The organization may also turn inward to educate and influence behaviors within its constituency and subject pool.

FIGURE 1

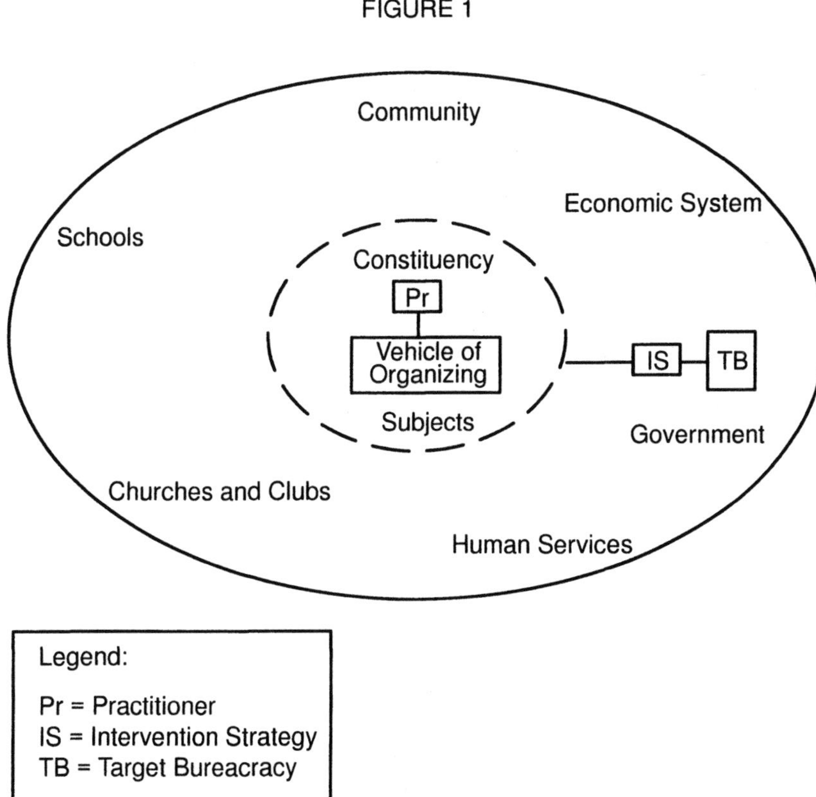

Legend:

Pr = Practitioner
IS = Intervention Strategy
TB = Target Bureacracy

MEMBERSHIP IN THE THREE MODALITIES

The pie chart, Figure 2, represents the sectors of the community which may be defined as parts of the constituency pool. The chart illustrates the context in which a cohesive commensalistic membership organization may be generated. Sectors represent functions or broad types of niches in the community. The center of the pie represents higher levels of stratification within a community; distance from the center represents lower status levels within the populations attached to the various functions.

Examining this figure, one can readily recognize that contrasting interests across the sectors and between status levels are likely to decrease the possibility of sustaining intense and cohesive commensalistic unions. Stated another way, diversity of status and function

FIGURE 2

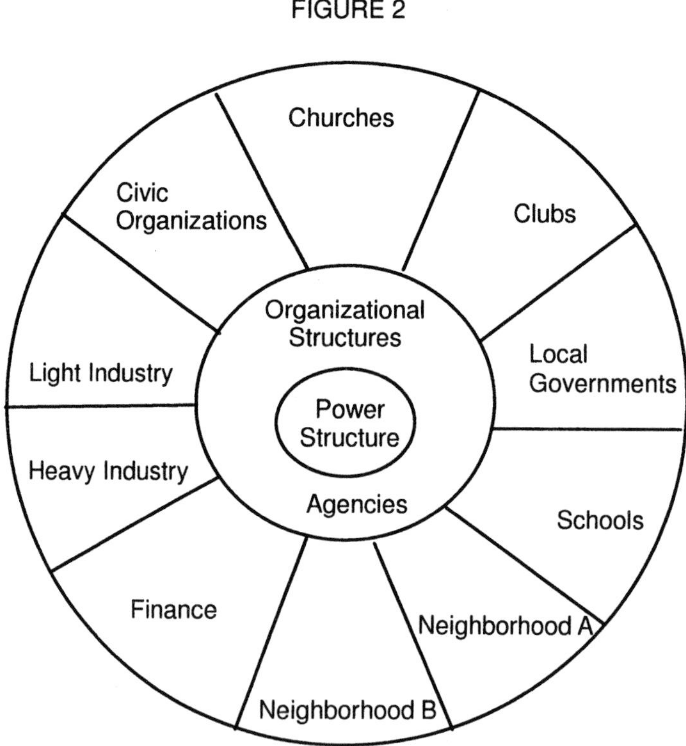

greatly reduces the likelihood of mutual identification with the stresses that sectional interest groups experience. On the other hand, homogeneity of status and function increases the likelihood of maintaining cohesion around a commonality of interest (Rogers, 1972).

The tasks of producing cohesion and achieving a consensus are different within each of these models. Taking the three modalities model of Cox, Erlich, Rothman, and Tropman (1974), members are drawn as follows:

1. traditional locality development–representatives from each sector and throughout the strata
2. socio-political action–representatives from one or more selected sectors, frequently from just one stratum within those sectors
3. social planning–representatives across sectors, within the near-elite strata

Locality Development

The problem with the ideal type of locality development is that representation is so diverse that little or no basis exists for commensalism. The common identity and problem must be stated so generally that they may hold little intense interest to such a broadly defined constituency, including sectors who feel exploited or disadvantaged by each other. The exceptions will be: (1) communities that are marginalized and disadvantaged as a whole, and (2) locality development memberships that are carefully selected to ignore sectional interests.

Socio-Political Action

A narrowly defined constituency more readily formulates its commensalism. Sectional and status interests can be well defined and may generate intense commitments to organizing, assuming the sense of collective efficacy has been developed. The goals of organizing and the life styles of members are more likely to coincide, and an intensity of self-expression is readily generated. Cohesion and solidarity are more readily built on a common identity.

Social Planning

Social planning bodies tend to be drawn from the well-educated, near elite and elite strata of a community. They may represent diverse functional sectors, but they communicate readily with one another, nevertheless. Their problem is a likelihood of confusion as to whose interests they represent. They frequently formulate their plans for "others." They combine motivations of helping those others, which may be perfectly sincere, with the self-interest of the elites in avoiding disruptive and embarrassing eruptions of criticism or disorder. Hence, social planning bodies tend to be well-regulated, even officious, thereby producing suspicion or resentment among their stated beneficiaries.

These are obviously ideal type models of community organization that may differ widely. Again, the principles are that: (1) stratification and functional diversity decrease the likelihood of sustaining intense and cohesive commensalistic unions, and (2) homogeneity increases the likelihood of maintaining cohesion. These principles have definite implications for the amount of energy that can be made available to a community organizing campaign.

THE THEORY OF HUMAN ENERGY CONSERVATION: AN ECOLOGICAL METAPHOR

The theory of the ecological practitioner requires first an understanding of the biological analogy. Earth and its minerals, water, air, and sunlight combine to provide the nutrients for living organisms. Each different form of living organism performs complex operations with these elements, transforming them into nutrients for further growth and development and generating byproducts which are used by other organisms as nutrients for other complex activities. Biochemists have determined that infinitesimal amounts of complex DNA molecules provide the signal and the transformational code for generative activities that feed further activities.

The organic byproducts of the ecosystem's dominant species may become symbiotic energy sources for a related species while, at the same time, these byproducts may impede the progress of other species. The theory of energy conservation suggests that energy is never lost. Instead, energy remains in the ecosystem by: (1) symbiotically providing nutrients to related organisms, (2) catalytically providing the genetic code that multiplies the energy sources for new activities, (3) cancelling the effect of nutrients for related organisms, or (4) dissipating into unreceptive environments where the potential energy rests unused for indefinite periods, called zero work in physics (Laue, 1950).

In the human ecosystem, any practitioner of community organization must assess the availability of human energy in response to the stimuli of the organizers. Whether by design or not, the organizers' actions may prove to be symbiotic, catalytic, impeding, or dissipating among the constituents and subjects they are designed to activate. In principle, each of these four responses can be anticipated as adaptations to the psychological, structural, political, socio-cultural, and economic frame of reference of various potential participants and affected sectors of the population.

The key point here is that the energy of the organizers is assumed to stimulate some kind of energy response. In fact, pressures of the situation, the style and socio-cultural fit of the organizers, and the timing predict the energy response. In the case of symbiosis, the energy response is summative. Catalytic stimulation is an energy multiplier. An impeding stimulus is negative. And a dissipating stimulus produces zero work.

Symbiosis

In the ecological perspective, social problems have been described as stressors for populations sectors which occupy disadvantaged niches in the community (Germain, 1985). To reduce the effects of these stressors, social planners or locality developers typically propose programs which offer some relief, such as day care for working mothers, job training and placement activities for the unemployed, parenting education for families of neglected children, mentoring activities for at-risk youth, and so on. These programs are shaped by individualized definitions of the stress to be relieved.

To the extent that these proposals offer net relief to people in stress, they fit the definition of stress reduction work. They can be expected to release and engender measured levels of energy among the sympathetic and grateful responses of the affected. Such programs are properly described as symbiotic: a need is met with some relief. An identified gap is filled with commensurate energy. Hence, participants in the organizing process can be expected to offer synergistic energy to the program, within the limits of the daily rhythms of their lives.

Catalytic Responses

On occasion, the pressures which cause personal suffering are identified as systematic in nature and a key system for overcoming the pressures is sought. The culture of the organizing effort includes the optimism that a key has been found which will achieve that goal. The organizers are seen by participants and the affected as the holders of that key. Their stimulus is timed, furthermore, to maximize the excitement of the response and the unleashing of energy. For its time, the War on Poverty of the 1960s was seen as such a catalyst, although it quickly deteriorated into a set of summative, routine programs. Certainly, the labor movement of the 1920s and 1930s, the civil rights movement of the 1950s and 1960s, the women's movement of the 1970s, and perhaps the gay and lesbian movement of the 1980s and 1990s are examples of social action catalysts. Energy was unleashed in multiplier fashion as their influence spread throughout the nation, altering American culture in their time and setting in motion catalytic responses which reached beyond the original stimulus through a series of iterations.

Impediments

Catalytic movements are known to produce backlashes. Sometimes, though not always, these reactive movements develop a legitimacy of their own among disaffected sectors who see the advantages of the movement to others as harmful to their status and life chances. In the ebb and flow of catalytic reactions, a well-intentioned organizer can become an impediment to the cause by setting in motion further reactions, without provoking the positive response among presumed followers. The socio-cultural explanations proposed by the organizer are not validated publicly. As a result, the stressors which cause suffering continue unabated and may become worse. The Lani Guinier episode in 1993 civil rights politics may serve as an example of this phenomenon.

Dissipated Energy

The energy of the organizers has been known to dissipate, producing zero work and making further positive efforts more difficult. Further energy for organizing is simply not available because of the loss of the dissipated energy. Organizers may assume that stressors are understood when they are not, or that participants are culturally attuned to the style of the organizer when they are not, or organizers may simply promote poor timing of the stimulus. Attempts by a social activist to embarrass community leaders when they are not embarrassed will ultimately produce dissipated energies among participants, for example. A community developer who insists on twice as many meetings as participants are willing to tolerate will likewise dissipate the expended energy. A social planner who incorrectly assesses the availability of funding resources may have a similar experience.

THE ENERGY ASSESSMENT

An effective practitioner will make an assessment of the projected available sources of human energy prior to designing and launching an organizing campaign. The energy assessment will take into account: (1) the centrality and saliency of the 'issue' and pent up energy among various projected participants, especially leaders, affected subjects, primary and secondary supporters, (2) the competing activities which may drain energy from those participants, both in the short run and the long run, (3) the participants' probable assessment of their opportunities for reward if goals are achieved, (4) the opportunities for association with like-minded people not otherwise available, (5) the efficacy of the action plan for achieving its goals, (6) the cultural acceptability to the participants of the style of action and the traditions of energy release, (7) the vulnerability of resistive targets, and (8) the likelihood that the leadership's credibility and inspiration can be undermined.

This assessment, of course, is highly subjective and the data gathering process is subjective. As such, it is susceptible to miscalculation. Organizers are not scientists whose predictions can be verified or quantified. Nevertheless, instances of similar organizing in other locations can be used as guides. The organizers must know themselves, their own commitment to the process, and their experience with potential participants.

SELECTION OF A STRATEGIC PATTERN OF ORGANIZING

Based on this assessment, practitioners may select different patterns of organizing, given the available energy among organizers and participants. One view of organizing focuses on its breadth. A narrow pattern is called pinpointing. This mode assumes that the available energy is minimal, but the balance of power in the negotiating arena favors the proponents even with minimal effort. A case in point would be a community program development campaign involving community entitlements which have summative effects.

In such a situation, energies can be conserved by involving few people in the organizing activity such as program developers and selected citizen spokespersons, limiting the number of organization meetings, and directing appointed agents to apply leverage, such as through a proposal. Organizers know, in this situation, that to expend their energy through broader patterns of organizing, in this situation, will be perceived as unnecessary and they will lose credibility. Likewise, if target resistance is expected while energies are unavailable, organizing efforts will fail and credibility will be lost.

The alternative broader pattern of organizing is called here voluminous organizing. This pattern assumes that the problem is widely salient and expanded fields of energy are available. It also assumes that resistance to the pleas of the proponents can be expected, thereby requiring potent and expanded uses of energy. "Expanded fields of energy" implies participation by broad classes of people in a catalytic campaign. The uses of energy might imply a key show of force through mass meetings, demonstrations, or more benign assemblies which are designed to represent a community consensus.

An application of the concept of energy to the steps of organizing produces strategic patterns of organizing as shown in Table 1 (adapted from MacNair, 1992).

Having calculated the total energy available for a given campaign, the practitioner must then determine how that energy will be most effectively distributed over the steps of organizing, allowing at least some of the steps to be handled in pinpoint fashion in order to conserve energy and save it for the critical moments of truth.

The theory of energy conservation assumes, then, that energy should be organized and spent in allotments that are commensurate with the energy assessment, high priority needs, and with the resistance expected. *Well timed, productive uses of energy are self-regenerating.* Misallocations of energy undermine one's own efforts. This is a proposition that is amenable to testing through empirical research. The theoretical proposition that is produced by this assumption may be stated as follows:

> *Voluminous expenditures of energy and resources for any step in a campaign which could have been achieved through pinpointing may reduce the energy available for each of the other steps in the campaign; pinpointing in this situation conserves energy, making it more available when it is needed. Pinpointed*

TABLE 1. Srategic Patterns and Steps of Organizing

	STRATEGIC PATTERNS OF ORGANIZING	
STEPS OF ORGANIZING	**PINPOINTED**	**VOLUMINOUS**
Organizational form	Mandated	Voluntary
Participation	Narrow	Extensive
Goals	Direct Service	Procedural
Needs assessments	Minimal data	Multiple forms
Inputs	Minimal	Extensive
Resource and policy negotiations	Few sources of support attempted	Many sources of support attempted

Adapted from MacNair, 1992.

expenditures of energy on high priority steps in which resistance is expected will likely result in failure, also lowering credibility and undermining the campaign; voluminous organizing in this situation is more likely to succeed, thereby increasing credibility.

PHASES OF ORGANIZING IN VARYING CAMPAIGN CIRCUMSTANCES

Further work is needed that discriminates between the preparatory phases of organizing (forming the group, gathering information and opinion, and forming a consensus) and the final leveraging phase in which strategies are applied to target organizations to achieve changes in policy or allocations of funds. The problem can be identified as *specification of the conditions which call for voluminous or pinpointing strategies in each of the two general phases (illustrated in Table 2).*

The Montgomery Bus Boycott of 1955 opened up new possibilities for civil rights campaigners. If discrimination on buses could be eliminated, all kinds of discrimination could be attacked. Extremely high levels of resistance were anticipated. To overcome this resistance, organizers knew that they must first demonstrate credible and strong cohesion within the aggrieved sector of the community. The preparatory task of identifying their problem and need and sustain-

TABLE 2. Phases and Strategic Patterns of Organizing in Different Types of Campaigns

PHASES	CAMPAIGN A	CAMPAIGN B	CAMPAIGN C	CAMPAIGN D
PREPARATION	VOLUMINOUS	VOLUMINOUS	PINPOINTED	PINPOINTED
LEVERAGING	VOLUMINOUS	PINPOINTED	VOLUMINOUS	PINPOINTED

Illustrations of the campaigns:

Campaign A: Montgomery bus boycott

Campaign B: Effort to be named a national demonstration site

Campaign C: Community education for child abuse

Campaign D: Planning for community entitlements

ing solidarity with that analysis required voluminous organizing. Even more so, the task of the leveraging phase, of convincing the bus company that demonstrators could consistently deprive them of their resources and reputation, required voluminous organizing. These highly intense and broad organizing campaigns were justified by the assumption of catalytic effects on American culture.

By contrast, the desire of a city to be named a national demonstration site in the National Cities Demonstration Act (Model Cities) required voluminous organizing in the preparatory phase, but not the leveraging phase (Campaign B). Federal guidelines which governed the application process required broad based involvement of various sectors of the community in legitimizing the structure, identifying problems, and forming a consensus backing the goals of the Demonstration Act.

Leveraging the grants, however, only involved specified elected officials and city administrators in the writing of the proposal, signing it, and transmitting it to the appropriate federal agency, a pinpointed organizing procedure. The summative nature of program outcomes belied the original justification that Model Cities programs would produce catalytic changes in the low income sectors of the community.

An example of pinpointed preparation and voluminous leveraging might be a community education campaign to educate teachers, parents, children, and neighbors about the signs of child abuse and its resolution (Campaign C). Pulling together a community task force, packaging the knowledge about child abuse and related procedures, and forming a consensus on goals can be handled in pinpointed fashion. The community education campaign, however, will require voluminous forms of outreach and involvement, including probably a broad-based volunteer corps of community educators. Opinions differ widely, however, on the catalytic or summative nature of such community education efforts.

Finally, a campaign to obtain funds for an interagency food program against hunger, assuming that the funds are a community entitlement (Campaign D), would be an example of a summative community practice involving both pinpointed preparation and leveraging. A selected network of agency and local governmental officials can perform the preparatory tasks, and another select set of volunteers and direct service workers can mobilize the food and administer it.

In summary, it can be said that a constitutive order governs the extent of involvement and the energy required in organizing both the preparatory and leveraging phases. Whether they are explicit and written or not, there are rules which can be discerned governing the kind of preparation needed and the nature of the organization required in the leveraging phase. Catalytic and summative assumptions distinctly appear to be involved in establishing this constitutive order.

COST, SPECIALIZATION, AND STYLE OF INTERVENTION

It may also be said that the nature of the goal or function itself is related to the level of investment in organizing. Hawley (1986) presents the theory of cost and functional specialization. In this theory, high costs in energy and resources reduce specialization and increase generality of function. In other words, a community organization campaign which targets broad, general gains for its constituency will require high expenditures of energy. Conversely, narrow specialization cannot be sustained in the face of high costs.

Styles of intervention can be identified and correlated with the degree of functional specialization in the campaign's target. For the sake of simplicity, it is assumed that intervention styles can be classified as either (1) nurturing and magnetic or (2) intrusive. Table 3 illustrates the dimensions of the two interventive strategies.

Nurturing strategies are based on an assumption that communication is the basic element needed to negotiate a desirable outcome. Communication is carried out with the intent to engage and persuade a target organization or population of the desired changes in policy or behavior. A shared set of values is assumed. Hence, strategies involving information and bonding are all that is required to strike a deal or effect a routine or technical change.

Intrusive strategies differ in that a shared set of values with the target is not assumed; some form of compulsion is needed to force compliance with the aims of the organized constituency. Communication may be startling and unexpected. Emotionally charged revelations are made which are evaluative or judgmental in nature.

TABLE 3

INTERVENTION STRATEGIES	DIMENSIONS OF INTERVENTION		
	RELATIONS	TRANSMISSION	CONTENT
Nurturing (magnetic)	bonding/ networking	normative/ educational	routine/ technical
Intrusive	punitive/ compelling	collective behavior	revelational/ evaluative

It is assumed here that intrusive strategies, which interfere with other people's business and policy and may require a change in the rules of decision-making, are energy-expensive. High levels of emotional energy are required; great efforts are required to mobilize the constituency for the campaign; and repercussions may give rise to further expenses. On the other hand, nurturant strategies, based on shared communication and affirmative bonding, are relatively inexpensive. Routine or technical messages do not require high levels of energy for organizing.

Combining the assumptions regarding energy and style of intervention with the proposition that energy cost correlates with functional generalization, it follows, as a theoretical proposition, that:

> *Intrusive strategies are expensive and will ultimately turn toward functionally general targets, including change in community norms. On the other hand, nurturant strategies are consistent with lower costs and specialized targets. A mismatch of strategies and targets will result in frustration and a change in either the strategy or the targets.*

Again, this statement can be tested empirically.

STYLES OF INTERVENTION AND STRATEGIC PATTERNS OF ORGANIZING

Finally, the two previous theoretical statements are interrelated. If the expenses of the strategy are related to the generality of the target and voluminous organizing is clearly more expensive, then it follows that:

> *Nurturant strategies may be effectively implemented through pinpointed patterns of organizing related to specialized targets, and intrusive strategies will tend to require voluminous patterns of organizing, related to generalized targets.*

An example of this last proposition is the civil rights movement of the 1950s and 1960s. The Montgomery bus boycott employed an intrusive strategy and voluminous modes of organizing, but its function was generalized over time. The initial goal was to alter the policy of segregating riders on buses, but the movement encountered the mass media and the basic assumptions of a segregated society. They accordingly broadened their targets, resulting ultimately in the Civil Rights Act of 1964 and the Voting Rights Act of 1965.

Nurturant strategies, on the other hand, relate a supplicant, for example, to a specialized authority target which controls resources. A pinpointed organizing pattern is adequate to reach such a target in most routine circumstances. Rape crisis centers, for example, typically employ a nurturing strategy and a pinpointed organizing pattern to affect the policies of police administrators.

CONCLUSION

Employing the proposed ecological theories of energy conservation and the strategic pattern of organizing, cost and specialization, and specialization and strategic pattern, it is possible to generate theory for practitioners which are amenable to empirical investigation, and practical in their scope.

Each of these theoretical propositions can be empirically tested and also demonstrated in practice just as Rothman did in his application studies (1976). Empirical research and demonstration will reveal exceptions, and those exceptions must be explained if the theory is to meet the evaluative criteria for good theory. Further refinement is required to produce a more complete theoretical construct for the ecological community practitioner.

This paper argues that ecological theory, with its focus on energy, is fertile ground for powerful theory building. Practitioners can use the if-then statements derived from the theoretical propositions discussed in this paper. Practitioners who embrace these theories can become theoreticians in their own practice.

REFERENCES

Bronfenbrenner, U. (1986). Ecology of the family as a context for human development: Research perspectives. *Developmental Psychology*, 22(6), 723-742.

Cook, K. (Ed.) (1987). *Social exchange theory.* Beverly Hills: Sage Publications.

Cox, F., Erlich, J., Rothman, J., & Tropman, J. (1974). *Strategies of community organization: A book of readings.* Itasca, IL: F.E. Peacock Publishers.

Gamson, W. A. (1975). *The strategy of social protest.* Homewood, IL: Dorsey Press.

Germain, C. (1985). The place of community work within an ecological approach to social work practice. In S. Taylor & R. Roberts (Eds.). *The theory and practice of community social work* (pp. 30-55). New York: Columbia University Press.

Hage, J. (1974). *Communication and organizational control: Cybernetics in health and welfare settings.* New York: John Wiley and Sons.

Hage, J. (1972). *Techniques and problems of theory construction in sociology.* New York: John Wiley and Sons.

Hage, J. (1981). *Theories of organizations: Form, process, and transformation.* New York: John Wiley and Sons.

Hawley, A. H. (1950). *Human ecology: A theory of community structure.* New York: Ronald Press.

Hawley, A. H. (1986). *Human ecology: A theoretical essay.* Chicago: University of Chicago Press.

Kahn, S. (1982). *Organizing.* New York: McGraw-Hill.

Laue, M. (1950). *History of physics.* New York: Academic Press.

Leiter, M., & Webb, M. (1983). *Developing human service networks.* New York: Irvington Publishers.

Long, N. (1962). *The polity.* Chicago: Rand McNally.

MacNair, R. (1992). Patterns of organizing for community human service planning: A statewide survey. In *Community organization and social administration: advances, trends, and emerging principles* (pp. 87-105). New York: The Haworth Press, Inc.

Martin, R., & Munger, P. (1962). *Decisions in Syracuse.* Bloomington, IN: Indiana University Press.

Meyer, C. (1983). *Clinical social work in the ecosystem perspective.* New York: University of Columbia Press.

Pecukonis, E., & Wenocur, S. (1994). The concept of individual and collective self efficacy in community organization theory and practice. *Journal of Community Practice*, 1(2).

Rogers, E. (1972). *Communication of innovations: A cross-cultural approach.* New York: The Free Press.

Rothman, J. (1974). *Planning and organizing for social change.* New York: Columbia University Press.

Rothman, J. (1976). *Promoting innovation and change in organizations and communities: A planning manual.* New York: Wiley and Sons.

Suttles, G. D. (1972). *The social construction of community.* Chicago: The University of Chicago Press.

Taylor, S., & Roberts, R. (1985). *The theory and practice of community social work.* New York: Columbia University Press.

Tropman, J. (1972). Comparative analysis of community organization agencies: The case of the welfare council. In I. A. Spergel (Ed.). *Community organization: Studies in constraint.* Beverly Hills, CA: Sage Publications.

Warren, R. (1963). *The community in America.* Chicago: Rand McNally and Company.

Warren, R. (1974). The structure of urban reform: Community decision organizations in stability and change. Lexington, MA: Lexington Books.

Waste, R. (1989). *The ecology of city policy making.* New York: Oxford University Press.

Index

Page numbers in italics indicate figures; page numbers followed by t indicate tables.

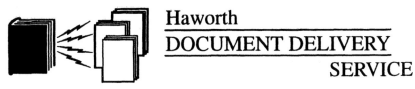

Haworth DOCUMENT DELIVERY SERVICE

This valuable service provides a single-article order form for any article from a Haworth journal.

- *Time Saving:* No running around from library to library to find a specific article.
- *Cost Effective:* All costs are kept down to a minimum.
- *Fast Delivery:* Choose from several options, including same-day FAX.
- *No Copyright Hassles:* You will be supplied by the original publisher.
- *Easy Payment:* Choose from several easy payment methods.

Open Accounts Welcome for . . .
- Library Interlibrary Loan Departments
- Library Network/Consortia Wishing to Provide Single-Article Services
- Indexing/Abstracting Services with Single Article Provision Services
- Document Provision Brokers and Freelance Information Service Providers

MAIL or *FAX* THIS ENTIRE ORDER FORM TO:

Haworth Document Delivery Service
The Haworth Press, Inc.
10 Alice Street
Binghamton, NY 13904-1580

or FAX: 1-800-895-0582
or CALL: 1-800-342-9678
9am-5pm EST

PLEASE SEND ME PHOTOCOPIES OF THE FOLLOWING SINGLE ARTICLES:

1) Journal Title: ______________________
Vol/Issue/Year: ____________ Starting & Ending Pages: ____________
Article Title: ______________________
____

2) Journal Title: ______________________
Vol/Issue/Year: ____________ Starting & Ending Pages: ____________
Article Title: ______________________
____

3) Journal Title: ______________________
Vol/Issue/Year: ____________ Starting & Ending Pages: ____________
Article Title: ______________________
____

4) Journal Title: ______________________
Vol/Issue/Year: ____________ Starting & Ending Pages: ____________
Article Title: ______________________
____

(See other side for Costs and Payment Information)

COSTS: Please figure your cost to order quality copies of an article.

1. Set-up charge per article: $8.00
   ($8.00 × number of separate articles) ________
2. Photocopying charge for each article:
   1-10 pages: $1.00 ________
   11-19 pages: $3.00 ________
   20-29 pages: $5.00 ________
   30+ pages: $2.00/10 pages ________
3. Flexicover (optional): $2.00/article ________
4. Postage & Handling: US: $1.00 for the first article/
   $.50 each additional article ________
   Federal Express: $25.00 ________
   Outside US: $2.00 for first article/
   $.50 each additional article ________
5. Same-day FAX service: $.35 per page ________

GRAND TOTAL: ____________

METHOD OF PAYMENT: (please check one)

❑ Check enclosed ❑ Please ship and bill. PO # ________________
(sorry we can ship and bill to bookstores only! All others must pre-pay)

❑ Charge to my credit card: ❑ Visa; ❑ MasterCard; ❑ Discover;
❑ American Express;

Account Number: ____________________ Expiration date: __________

Signature: ✗ ________________________________

Name: ____________________ Institution: ____________________

Address: ____

____

City: ____________________ State: ________ Zip: __________

Phone Number: ________________ FAX Number: ________________

MAIL or *FAX* THIS ENTIRE ORDER FORM TO:

Haworth Document Delivery Service	**or FAX:** 1-800-895-0582
The Haworth Press, Inc.	**or CALL:** 1-800-342-9678
10 Alice Street	9am-5pm EST)
Binghamton, NY 13904-1580